THE DEVELOPMENT OF A MEDICINE

In all experimental knowledge there are three
phases : An observation is made, a comparison
is established and a judgment rendered.

C. Bernard (1865)

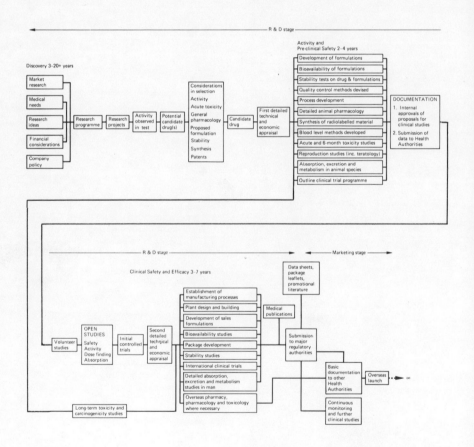

Stages in the discovery and development of a typical drug (courtesy ICI and the *Financial Times*).

THE DEVELOPMENT
OF A
MEDICINE

R. B. Smith

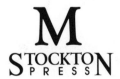

M
STOCKTON PRESS

First published 1985

Published in the United Kingdom by
THE MACMILLAN PRESS LTD
Houndmills, Basingstoke, Hampshire RG21 2XS
and London
Companies and representatives
throughout the world

Printed in Hong Kong

British Library Cataloguing in Publication Data
Smith, Richard B.
The development of a medicine.
1. Pharmacology
I. Title
615'.1   RM300
ISBN 0-333-36884-3
ISBN 0-333-36885-1 Pbk

Published in the United States and Canada by
Stockton Press
15 East 26th Street, New York, NY 10010

Library of Congress Cataloging in Publication Data
Smith, R. B. (Richard Barry), 1940–
    The development of a medicine.
    1. Pharmacy. 2. Pharmacy—Research. 3. Drugs—
Testing. 4. Drug trade. I. Title. [DNLM: 1. Clinical
Trials. 2. Drug Evaluation. 3. Drug Industry.
4. Research. QV 771 S657d]
RS92.S63 1985   615'.7   85–4780
ISBN 0-943818-09-5

To Stephanie, Edward, Alexander and William

Contents

alternative synthetic substances. 'Molecular roulette' synthesis. Early animal testing. Pilot batch manufacture. Establishment of specifications. Scale-up. The assurance of quantity and quality of the material

Biological   32

Pharmacological investigations into primary and secondary effects in animals and organ systems in both normal and abnormal models. Isolated-organ work. Intention and aspiration to give predictability of effects in man. Studies of absorption, distribution, metabolism and excretion in animals after single and multiple dosing

4   SAFETY EVALUATION (ANIMAL STUDIES)   45

Build-up of knowledge from LD 50 studies through 7-day, 3-month and 12-month toxicity studies in a number of different species. Fertility testing, peri- and post-natal studies. Teratology, mutagenicity and carcinogenicity testing

5   FORMULATION DEVELOPMENT   53

Development of various types of injections, and irritation studies. Advantages and disadvantages of different tablet and capsule presentations. Common problems with some formulations. Sugar coating and film coating. Syrups, suspensions, ointments, creams, suppositories, pessaries, implants, powders and aerosols, etc. Stability testing. Product security and child safety

6   HUMAN PHARMACOLOGY   63

Volunteer studies. Human pharmacokinetics — absorption, distribution, metabolism and excretion studies. Preparation of volunteers and conduct of trials. Dose–effect relationships. Steady-state kinetics. Single- and multiple-dosage investigations. Bioavailability studies — alternate formulations. Special investigations. Discussion of true and false positives and negatives in both pharmacology and toxicology

Foreword

Medicines, and the drugs they contain, are taken for granted by most people. We have been born and bred in a generation whose medicine cabinets contain 'something for every occasion' — analgesics for pain, antacids for indigestion, laxatives for constipation, contraceptives, and, all too often, antidepressants, tranquillisers and sleeping pills. So conditioned have we become to thinking that 'there is a pill for every problem' that many of us forget the equally important truism 'every pill has its problem and its price'.

The price of a drug is not only the enormous cost of its development, assessment and marketing, but also the sum of adverse effects which it may inflict, and which have to be accepted by the few if its beneficial effects are to be enjoyed by the many. We cannot be reminded too often of this risk–benefit ratio which every therapeutically active medicine possesses, and in this book Dr Smith spells out the situation clearly and concisely, based on his long experience in drug development.

An understanding of the processes that lead to the discovery of new medicines and the balanced assessment of their therapeutic roles may lead to a better appreciation of their true value and a more responsible approach to their use. This is essential if the true potential of drug treatment is to be realised in the conquest of disease.

Paul Turner
Professor of Clinical Pharmacology
St Bartholomew's Hospital
London, EC1

Preface

This book has been in gestation for almost five years. During this time I have been made aware repeatedly of the fact that, although many people do have a genuine interest in how their medicines come into being, relatively few have an overall view on how this development of a medicine is achieved. Therefore the major purpose of this book is to provide a general 'broad-brush' impression of the many components of drug development. It aims to draw together and associate the various disciplines which interrelate and interact to make the end result — a safe and effective medicine for human use — a reality.

Goring-on-Thames, 1985   *R.B.S.*

Acknowledgments

I would like to record my sincere thanks to the many friends, both in 'academia' and industry, who, by their advice and encouragement have helped me in writing this book. My especial thanks are due also to Dr Eric Cliffe, Dr Desmond Fitzgerald and Professor Kenneth Bentley who have given their time to render essential practical assistance by providing significant amounts of illustrative material, and to Mrs M. J. Wyburn-Mason for kind permission to use part of illustration number 24a from *The Causation of Rheumatoid Disease and Many Human Cancers*. The Royal Society of Medicine has also been most helpful in locating and photographing illustrative material.

I am extremely grateful for the forbearance, patience and accuracy of Sarah Tobitt and Carol Miller who typed the manuscript through its various drafts and revisions.

1
Introduction

Since nearly everyone takes medicines at some stage in their lives and often with some frequency, the development of medicines should be of concern to all. Originally they were made in small quantities from natural substances and the compounding of such remedies suffered from the obvious defect that standardisation both by the same doctor on different occasions, and between different doctors, was impossible. Furthermore, until relatively recent times the compounding, dispensing and administration of medicinals was associated with varying degrees of magic.

Even over the last one hundred years the invention and development of medicines has continued to be shrouded in mystery. Where it is not shrouded in mystery it is largely taken for granted, since public interest is usually only aroused by the modern-day media in the latter stages, either when the medicine becomes available for use by the general public and is hailed as an advance, or is associated with a real or exaggerated catastrophe.

Commencing really with the Thalidomide disaster, public interest and awareness in the safety of medicines has recently increased, and this has been latterly reinforced by the situation surrounding the withdrawal from world markets of both benoxaprofen (Opren) and, to a lesser extent, zomepirac (Zomax). Although the Thalidomide disaster resulted in increased legislative activity and control, both this and later events have done little to uncloak the process whereby a new developmental medicine is eventually shown to be safe and effective for use by man, and introduced to the prescriber. Therefore the purpose of this book is to present a vignette of how medicines are derived and to outline what happens to them in the ten years or so that they may be in development before they are eventually released for general use by the family doctor. The process whereby this is achieved is extremely complex and to be successful depends upon a high level of integration between specialists drawn from vastly dissimilar scientific disciplines within the pharmaceutical industry, often leavened with a cross-fertilisation of ideas and co-operation from university scientists, clinicians and other personnel.

As it happens, the vast majority of significant developments have arisen as a result of investment both in time and materials by private companies. Some

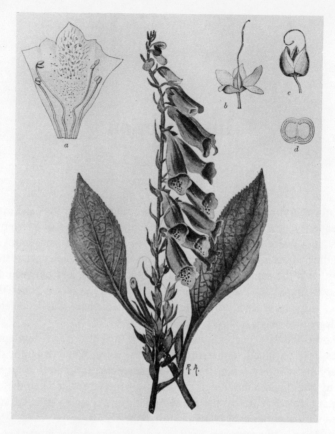

Figure 1   The major features of recognition of the poisonous foxglove (*Digitalis purpurea*) are shown in this plate from Strasburger's *Text-book of Botany* (1930). For many years the cardiac drug digitalis was prepared from the leaves either dried or used as a 'tea'. It is not surprising that standardisation of potency was impossible and therapeutic effects diffcult to predict. Eventually potency was standardised and the drug prepared as Digoxin.

companies have been extremely successful, others less so. Even those which have enjoyed success seem to exhibit it in a phasic fashion and often go through long fallow periods.

Superficially at any rate, this success appears to be determined by a critical personality mix coupling an effective innovative capability with other specialists whose interests and talents lie in piloting the substance through the 'mine field' which is development. Although the process is commonly called *development*, it is in fact *research*, using as the definition for this word 'the seeking for and interpretation of new knowledge'. Each new compound pursues an individual course of development. If this were not so and products could be developed by a 'manual', many more companies would be much more effective at producing new medicines in faster timescales.

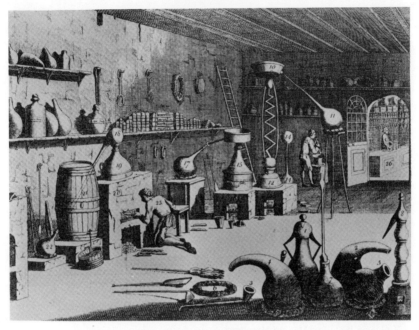

Figure 2 An eighteenth-century manufactory of drugs with a direct sales outlet to the public (far right). This establishment was probably more well-ordered than most but obviously any 'batch-to-batch' control of the products would have been impossible even if the need had been appreciated. (Line engraving published for the Universal Magazine, 1747 – impression in the Wellcome Historical Medical Museum.)

COMPONENT PARTS OF DEVELOPMENT

This account has been divided into various sections in an attempt to break down this complicated integrated process into a number of readily identifiable steps. However, the steps do not necessarily proceed sequentially. Often they occur coincidentally although their rates of progress may vary. The need therefore for an effective 'team effort' is self evident if success is to be achieved. The major stages in drug development, which will be examined in more detail below, are:

- Discovery
- Basic scientific characterisation:
    1. Chemical
    2. Biological
- Safety evaluation (animal studies)
- Formulation development
- Human pharmacology
- Evaluation of human efficacy and safety
- The regulatory process

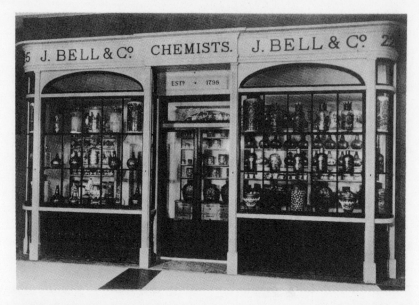

Figure 3   In contrast to the manufactory, the well-ordered and sophisticated public aspect
of the apothecary's business is seen in this view of the reconstructed facade of Bell's shop in
the Wellcome Historical Medical Museum.

- Marketing
- Project co-ordination
- Manufacture and supply
- The post-registration phase
- International development

While all of the above steps, which are broadly sequential, are proceeding,
further specialised work (starting from the basic characterisation of the new
medicine) is in train. In the main this is directed towards ensuring an adequate
supply of the medicine of an acceptable degree of *purity*, which is then developed into a formulation to ensure the medicine reaches the parts of the body it
is designed to affect in adequate *quantity* and at the right *time*. Therefore there
is an additional process which is critical. This is chemical process development,
often leading on to eventual large-scale production. Interlocked with it is formulation design and development. Ideally the final formulation should be established as early as possible, since the attainment of comparability in clinical
pharmacology, and subsequent clinical investigational work, depends upon the
early availability of an acceptable formulation.

Therefore the whole rationale for the above schema is to ensure that the
medicine is what it is supposed to be, that it does not contain harmful con-
taminants, and that it is given in the right dose and at the right time in order to
produce a predictable and desired effect.

It follows therefore that unacceptable unwanted effects should not arise. However, all active medicines produce some unwanted effects, but it is a question of degree. The balance between good effects and bad is called the *therapeutic ratio* and, of course, this can vary in different situations. This will be examined in more detail later.

DEVELOPMENT COSTS

So far the cost of developing a new medicine has not been considered. Over the past twenty years costs have risen enormously, from approximately £500,000 in the later 1950s and early 1960s to anything between £10,000,000 and £30,000,000 at 1984 prices, the actual cost depending on the complexity of the medicine being developed. Of course, a certain amount of this difference is due to inflation, but even when corrected for inflation the figures show a steady rise. This has been brought about as a direct result of events such as the Thalidomide episode which has increased the demand by the legislators for more control over the development of medicines in the hope that absolute safety can be achieved. This demand has led in turn to more complex animal testing and the maintenance of some of these tests for a longer period of time. These factors have added to the cost not just in terms of the costs of the animals involved, but also those costings directly attributable to the people who look after the animals, clean them and feed them, and operate the facilities required to house them for long periods of time. Then there is the critically important work involved in preparing and inspecting many thousands of specimens generated from these animals. Added to this is the huge volume of paperwork created as a result which has to be managed. All of these factors conspire together so that not only are medicines more expensive to develop but also they take much longer from the stage of discovery to their eventual release for use by the doctor. Clinical studies have also increased both in terms of time and complexity in this effort to quantify the truth.

Reviewing the events of the last two decades it has become increasingly apparent that the search for absolute safety for each and every individual is like pursuing the Holy Grail. The most important thing to bear in mind at all stages in the development and use of a medicine is the therapeutic ratio. The interpretation of this is of course a matter of judgement and must be related to the circumstances existing at every individual application of the medicine.

DEVELOPMENT TIME-SPAN

Whereas twenty years ago the average time for development was of the order of two to four years, this has now increased to an average of at least eight years and if the required animal and human work is extremely complex, it can last much longer. However it is true to say that much much more is known about a medicine nowadays before it comes on to the market than was hitherto the case.

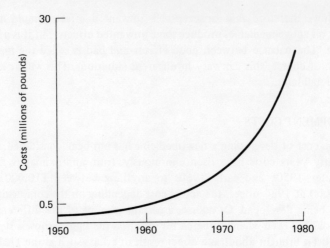

Figure 4 The cost of developing new medicines has risen inexorably over the last 30 years as a result of increased animal and human testing, in turn arising from increasingly exacting regulatory requirements.

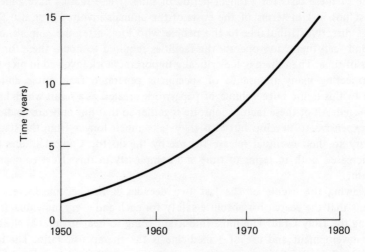

Figure 5 The increase in total possible development time, from about two years in 1950 to fifteen or more years in 1980, is related to the increased developmental work required to satisfy regulations and the difficulty of identifying new advances in therapy.

SUCCESS RATE

It has been estimated that on average only one compound in 10,000 is capable of successful development into a medicine used widely by man. It is always difficult to substantiate such a figure but of course it seeks to take into consideration all of those drugs that fail at different stages of investigation. Normally the majority 'bite the dust' early on. Those that make it through into human testing become more and more likely to be capable of development into human medicines as the pathway proceeds. However, as we shall see, even in the late stages of clinical testing or even indeed following successful marketing, a drug may reveal unsuspected and unacceptable human toxicity which could lead to restriction of prescribing or even its immediate withdrawal from use.

2
Discovery

From ancient times, man, by a process of trial and error, has identified a number of plants and other substances which either eaten raw or boiled up will produce certain pharmacological effects. The classic example is probably alcohol which virtually every culture learned to produce independently. Alcohol has a number of well-known effects depending upon the dosage used. In small amounts it causes flushing of the skin (vasodilatation), larger quantities produce a feeling of well-being, and if the dose is further increased, loss of inhibition occurs leading to signs of aggression. Beyond aggression, somnolence occurs and indeed coma can supervene as the central nervous system becomes progressively depressed. This well-known continuum of effects illustrates very neatly the effect of increasing dosage over a period of time with a substance which is metabolised simply and at a fairly constant rate. It further illustrates that where small quantities of a drug are useful, larger quantities are not necessarily better, in fact they are usually harmful.

The good or harmful properties of various other materials were also discovered by trial and error (coca leaves – cocaine; poppy juice – opium, containing approximately 9-17% of morphine) by many cultures.

However, the practice of medicine remained more or less in this rudimentary form up until quite recent times, when in the seventeenth and eighteenth centuries certain other therapeutic effects began to be realised.

PREVENTION OF SCURVY

Although scurvy, the deficiency state induced by a lack of fresh vegetables and fruit, had been known for centuries, it was not until the development of the long sea voyages of discovery from the sixteenth century onwards that the importance of this condition in reducing the efficiency, and eventually the numbers, of a ship's crew came to be appreciated. During the course of what is now acknowledged as probably the first recorded controlled clinical trial, Lind in 1747 identified that the administration of lemon juice was specific in relieving the symptoms of scurvy. However, it took another 53 years before the administration of lemon juice to the crews of Royal Navy ships was declared

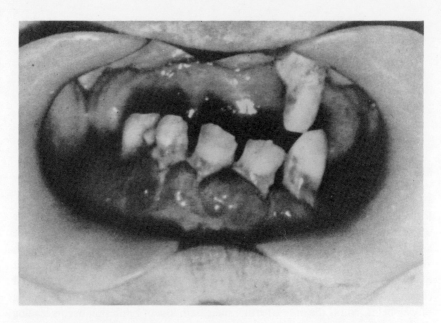

Figure 6   The bleeding, pulpy gums characteristic of scurvy (vitamin C deficiency) which progresses to infection and loss of the teeth(courtesy John Marks, *A Guide to Vitamins*, 1975).

compulsory. During the course of the nineteenth century a flirtation with lime juice for commercial reasons ensured the reappearance of the condition until it was realised that limes contain about half as much Vitamin C as lemons. The reason it occurs at all is that man (together with monkeys and guinea pigs) is distinct from other mammals in that he cannot synthesise Vitamin C. To maintain health it therefore has to be obtained from a food source and this is normally satisfactorily supplied by fresh fruit and vegetables.

Ascorbic Acid or Vitamin C was chemically characterised during the early 1930s and nowadays additionally required supplies are manufactured by chemical synthesis.

TREATMENT OF MALARIA

Following the Spanish conquest of South America the bark of the Cinchona was recognised as a remedy for malaria. Named Peruvian or Jesuits' bark it was shipped to Europe in quantity and by the mid-seventeenth century was acknowledged as a remedy in contemporary continental medical literature, appearing in the London Pharmacopoeia in 1677. By 1820 Pelletier and Caventou had isolated quinine and cinchonine from the bark which contains about 2% of quinine-type alkaloids. In contrast to that of Vitamin C, quinine synthesis is complex and until it was superseded by other anti-malarials, quinine was obtained from natural sources. Its chemistry is interesting since it has been shown that the chemical (secondary alcohol) grouping connecting the two major parts of the molecule is essential for anti-malarial activity and appears to create a suitable balance between efficacy and toxicity. Now replaced by chemically synthesised anti-malarials, quinine has contributed to our understanding of the therapeutic activity of this type of compound.

RELIEF OF PAIN AND INFLAMMATION

Also known for centuries (used by Hippocrates fourth century BC and described by Galen in the second century AD) was the medicinal effect of willow bark definitively described by the Reverend Edmund Stone in the mid-eighteenth century, and its bitter glycoside called Salicin (after Salix — willow) was identified by Leroux in 1827. The acid derivative was soon synthesised and by 1860 had been manufactured from phenol in Germany. The sodium salt was used for rheumatic fever in 1875 by Buss and this observation was independently confirmed by Stricker and MacLagan in 1879. Its effect in alleviating symptoms of gout (by increasing excretion of the accumulating uric acid) was identified in the same year. Within twenty years, acetylsalicylic acid (aspirin) which had been discovered in 1863 was introduced into medicine to control both pain and inflammation and as an antipyretic by Hoffmann of Bayer in 1897. Despite the recent vast increase of synthesised anti-inflammatory agents of many different structures, aspirin has, in the opinion of many, never been bettered. Current worldwide consumption of aspirin in various forms is of the order of thousands of tonnes.

CARDIAC MEDICINE

Similarly digitalis (from foxglove — see figure 1) and other plant extracts with an action on the heart have been known for centuries, but it was not until 1785 when William Withering wrote his famous treatise that its effect on oedema (dropsy) was definitely described. Later writers (Ferriar) emphasised the effect of digitalis on the heart. After much indiscriminate use in the nineteenth century, digitalis became established in the treatment of both atrial fibrillation and congestive cardiac failure during the twentieth century as the subtleties of its various actions came to be realised, often as the result of trial and error.

These few substances, opium (for its anti-diarrhoeal as well as pain-relieving properties), Vitamin C, Jesuits' bark and digitalis were in reality the hard core of the physicians' armamentarium by the close of the eighteenth century. Of course they were supplemented by various mixtures, tinctures and potions which were of unsubstantiated medicinal value.

As the nineteenth century wore on, two major advances arose in the form of antiseptic surgery (Lister and his carbolic acid spray) which was facilitated by the use of anaesthetic agents, both general (ether and chloroform) and local (cocaine). Although real advances, these did not benefit the average doctor to any great extent in his day-to-day practice of medicine.

SELECTIVITY

However, in the 1870s Ehrlich in the course of his research noted the specificity of certain dyes for certain tissues. Out of this was born the concept of selectivity, that is that the possibility might exist to destroy micro-organisms and parasites while leaving host tissues relatively unaffected. As a result arsphenamine (Salvarsan — Ehrlich's magic bullet) was developed and this was later improved upon with neosalvarsan which was used until the early 1940s. By the close of the nineteenth century pure aspirin as an analgesic and anti-inflammatory agent had become available and shortly after that the barbiturate group of drugs represented by phenobarbitone was employed in the treatment of epilepsy.

Reviewing matters at the beginning of the nineteenth century it is apparent that the therapeutic revolution and later explosion was off to a very slow start indeed. Apart from advances in the actual practice of surgery already noted, the physician's armamentarium had been supplemented only by an anti-infective agent of relatively low potency, a non-narcotic (non-opium derived) analgesic — aspirin — and a central nervous system depressing agent — phenobarbitone.

CHEMICAL RESEARCH

The next major development was that of the sulphonamides but this was a long and painful gestation indeed and the prototype compound prontosil red as a bacteriostatic (as opposed to bactericidal) agent did not appear until 1935.

Eventually this was very much improved upon with the preparation of sulphapyridine (M and B 693) which was successfully used to treat the late Sir Winston Churchill in World War II. Still following this line of anti-microbial attack, in 1928, as many readers will know, Fleming made a chance observation which was to permit the identification and development of penicillin which freed humanity for the first time from the ever-present dangers of intercurrent infection. Fleming's discovery was not really capitalised upon until the war years when the techniques of production of penicillin in quantity by fermentation were hurriedly developed. Initially penicillin was available for use only by injection (benzyl penicillin — Penicillin G). This was followed by the development of procaine penicillin which was a long-acting preparation, and by 1950 Penicillin V for oral administration was available. The years since the mid-1950s have seen an explosion in the availability of different forms of penicillin where the object has been to combat constantly developing resistance of the adaptable bacteria and also to extend the spectrum of activity of this class of compound to kill different strains and types.

Following the advent of oral penicillin, various penicillinase-producing staphylococci which were able to destroy penicillin were identified. These were

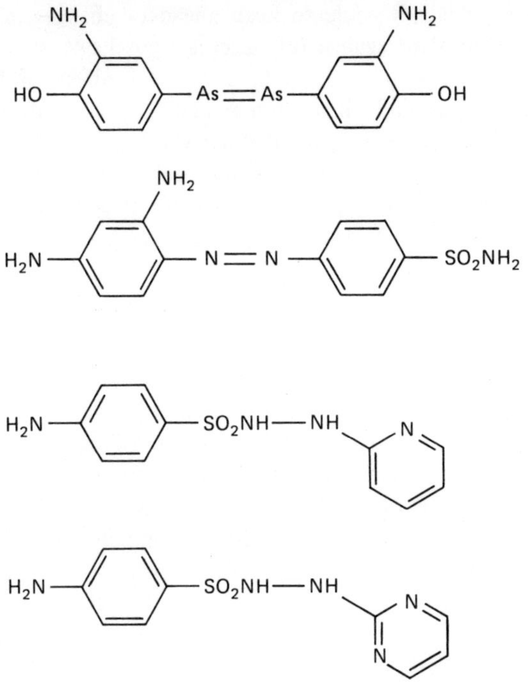

Figure 7 The structural similarities between arsphenamine, Prontosil (the red dye), sulpha-pyridine and sulphadiazine can be seen. However, these seemingly similar chemicals have significantly differing potentials for toxicity.

counteracted by methicillin (which could overcome bacterial penicillinase). This was available for parenteral use only. Inevitably oral penicillins of this type followed when protection of the beta-lactam ring was achieved. These isoxazolyl penicillins suffered from the drawback of a narrow spectrum of action. However, in 1957 the basic penicillin core was isolated, identified and prepared in a pure crystalline form. This was 6-aminopenicillanic acid. Subsequent developments have essentially been to manipulate and substitute on the side chain of the acid core. Therefore the production of penicillin has advanced from a laborious fermentation process to a semi-synthetic and finally a fully synthetic procedure. Apart from ease of manufacture it has permitted a standardisation of the product. Two other major developments in the fight against infection should not be forgotten. One was the isolation of streptomycin in 1944 and the second was the development of tetracyclines in the late 1940s. Both of these early development are still used in the control of infections like tuberculosis and tetracycline also for other less serious respiratory conditions. However, bacteria as a group are both tenacious and versatile and the fight against infection is still proceeding.

Most recent developments have been the cephalosporins first in parenteral and latterly in oral form (cephalexin) and future research will no doubt seek to modify the basic bactericidal molecule to keep ahead of changes in bacterial resistance. The story of the fight against infection is a good one as it illustrates first of all the need for continuous development to 'stay ahead of the game' (*vis-à-vis* the bacteria) and secondly how commercialisation of a product on a wide scale not only makes it available to all those who could benefit from its use, but also brings in its train production on a large scale and at greatly reduced cost. The cost in time and effort in producing a gram of penicillin nowadays is miniscule and in stark contrast to the costs incurred during the early 1940s.

BIOLOGICAL RESEARCH

Turning aside from this pathway of chemical-based development aimed at combating infections we must return to the late nineteenth and early twentieth century which witnessed a vast increase in the amount of biological research and enquiry. Central to this particular struggle is the story of diabetes which was momentously researched by Banting and Best in the early 1920s. Starting from relatively simple replacement therapy, diabetics have been managed using various naturally produced insulins which over the years have been refined in terms of potency and duration of action. Because of the natural origin of the material many difficulties such as allergic reactions have been experienced in the treatment of these patients. However, recent developments in micro-biological production of pure insulin have set some of these problems aside. During the 1920s and 1930s the accent was on replacement therapy for certain conditions. Apart from insulin there were thyroid extracts and pancreatic extracts, and the role of Vitamin B_{12} in pernicious anaemia was recognised.

THE RECOGNITION OF STRESS

In the late 1940s Hans Selye published his treatise on stress, and whereas compound E (cortisone) had been isolated in 1935 it was only synthesised in 1948. The molecule was later substantially chemically modified to produce the synthetic steroids prednisone and prednisolone in the early 1950s. This offered new hope for those with rheumatoid arthritis and similar inflammatory disorders. The compounds were also found to benefit asthma sufferers and steroids as topical preparations also brought relief from itching and inflammation to those with eczema and allied disorders. However, the use of these steroid compounds for any appreciable length of time was soon recognised to be accompanied by unacceptable side effects. Based upon the well-known properties of aspirin, a search then began for non-steroidal anti-inflammatory agents which it was hoped would have the advantages of the steroid compounds but without the concomitant disadvantages. This line of research pursued by many different companies has now resulted in an enormous range of these compounds, and where none can be said to give absolute relief of the condition in terms of either

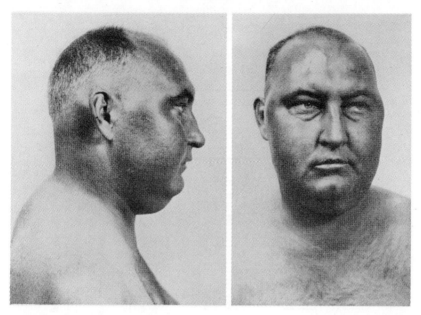

Figure 8 Cushing's disease. Excessive administration of steroids produces untoward deposition of fat, fluid retention and skin pigmentation. This occurred when these agents were used to control conditions such as eczema and asthma and before the untoward effects were appreciated. (From Cushing, H. (1932). Besophil adenomes of the pituitary body, *Bull. Johns Hopkins Hosp.*, Vol. L, 179.)

halting or reversing rheumatoid disease, they nonetheless have made a signal contribution to the quality of life of thousands of people.

SELECTIVITY REVISITED

About the same time, Alquist (1948) enunciated his receptor theory where he stated that the actions of noradrenalin in the body were mediated through designated alpha and beta receptors. Whereas the action of noradrenalin on alpha receptors produced vasoconstriction with an increase in blood pressure, dilatation of the pupils and gut relaxation, the action of this chemical on beta receptors produced an increase in cardiac output by enhancing cardiac excitability and increasing its rate of beating. Beta receptors also mediated arterial dilatation and bronchial relaxation. The actual results therefore of a noradrenalin injection seen in intact man was a combination or interaction of all of these different effects. Since the early years the receptor theory has advanced and has been refined. It is now recognised that there are $alpha_1$ (post-synaptic) receptors which are responsible for excitation and vaso-constriction. There are in addition $alpha_2$ (pre-synaptic) receptors which represent a 'cut off' mechanism and inhibit noradrenalin release by negative feedback. Considering the beta side, there are $beta_1$ receptors which mediate the effect of noradrenalin on the heart

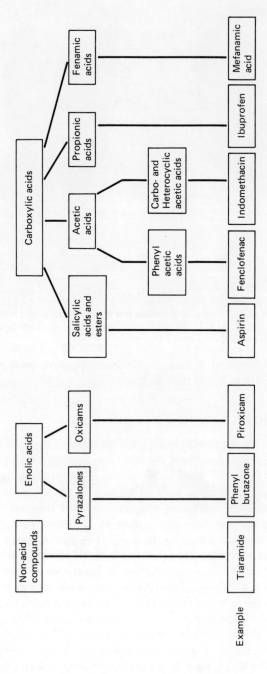

Figure 9 Non-steroidal anti-inflammatory compounds. The components of this major group of therapeutically active compounds are shown here. All are effective to differing degrees and toxicity also varies. Although fenclofenac and phenylbutazone have recently been withdrawn because of toxicity, ibuprofen, on the other hand is considered safe enough to be sold, like aspirin, to the public without a doctor's prescription but under a pharmacist's control.

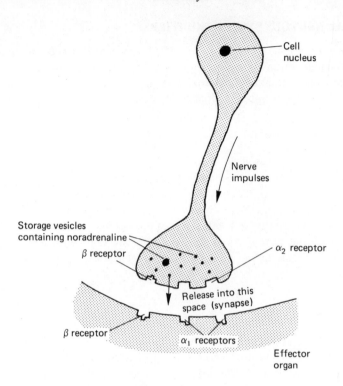

Figure 10 The receptor theory. Basically, a nerve impulse going down a nerve to its ending produces release of noradrenaline, which will have different effects depending on which receptor it becomes attached to – e.g. β_1 (heart), β_2 (lungs), α_1 various body sites and α_2 (the nerve cell itself). This last is important because it represents a 'cut-off' mechanism preventing further release of noradrenaline. Receptors work on a 'lock-and-key' principle. Thus medicines which are designed to enhance, block or otherwise modify this system must resemble noradrenaline in some degree so that they will fit the lock (see figure 11).

and beta$_2$ receptors governing effects on the lungs. On this basic theory and its subsequent refinements and modifications is founded the development since the mid-1950s of anti-hypertensive therapy. Different companies have pursued different lines with the result that there is now a wide variety of anti-hypertensive agents operating on alpha receptors either centrally (in the brain) or peripherally at pre- and post-synaptic sites (α-receptor blockade). Alternatively, beta-receptor blockade, which affects the heart's action, may be used. Nor does it end there since beta blockers have been found useful in controlling various disorders of cardiac rhythm and in cutting down cardiac work to bring relief to suffers from angina pectoris. Recent work, in contrast, has concentrated on the renal angio-tensin system and calcium metabolism to combat the progress of hypertension.

The three lines of research and development so far described (anti-infectives, non-steroidal anti-inflammatory agents and cardiovascular modifying agents) might be said to be enough in themselves. However the story goes further.

CENTRAL NERVOUS SYSTEM MODIFIERS

In the 1940s various agents were identified which had effects on the central nervous system. From these observations has stemmed an enormous variety of major and minor tranquillisers, anxiolytic and hypnotic agents together with treatments for Parkinsonism (L-dopa) and advances in the treatment of epilepsy.

POPULATION CONTROL

In addition, society has been radically changed by the development of oral contraceptives. Originally the emphasis was quite rightly on efficacy, but as usage and experience increased it became well-recognised that oestrogen/progesterone combinations in certain doses were associated with rare but often drastic unwanted effects. Since the 1960s this area too has been the subject of constant attention with the current development of effective oral contraceptive preparations which contain lower amounts of oestrogen and progesterone than ever before.

ANTI-CANCER

Although it is something of a Cinderella in terms of pharmaceutical development, the development of cytotoxic agents in the fight against cancer should not be forgotten. Because of these developments, certain types of cancer are now susceptible of cure or very-long-term remission. The difficulty has been, and still is, that of fully utilising Ehrlich's magic bullet concept. That is to say, the development of agents which will selectively kill abnormal cells wherever they are in the body but which will not significantly affect normal healthy cells. Much recent work has concentrated on utilising the body's own selective protection/destruction system mediated through its immune response to achieve this end.

RECENT MAJOR DEVELOPMENTS

Finally in recording this explosion in therapeutic development which has taken place virtually only in the last thirty-five years, mention must be made of two recent further utilisations of the receptor theory.

Firstly the development of histamine (H_2) receptor antagonists, which by their action in blocking the production of gastric acid, have led for the first time to effective control of active gastric and duodenal ulceration. This development has brought significant relief to many thousands of sufferers from peptic ulceration.

Secondly in terms of relief from misery has been the intense search for an ideal analgesic. Current opinion holds that this should have all the good characteristics of morphine but without the drawbacks, and many companies have expended vast sums in this search. Recently with the identification of natural analgesic substances (enkephaline) the receptor theory has been invoked again. As the characteristics of receptors become more and more completely quantified then the possibility of development of more suitable analgesics is envisaged.

It is difficult to summarise the progress of therapeutics in relatively few words and the above account omits to mention many important offshoots of development such as the development of oral anti-diabetic and early diuretic agents stemming from sulphonamide research. However, the above account is intended to show that research and development is very much a question of progress, often painstakingly achieved, almost like a sound wave with a hemispherical wave front. The most important part of this process is the creation of 'enabling science'. That is to say, all those seemingly unrelated observations which have to be made before someone comes along and with a flash of inspiration puts the whole jigsaw together. Indeed the mere act of fitting some of the pieces together, however imperfectly, will spark off other individuals to complete the pattern.

It has been said recently that the process of drug discovery and development has become much more difficult because 'we have run out of the basic science'. Nothing in fact could be further from the truth. The frontier of basic knowledge where vastly dissimilar disciplines interlock is continually being pushed back. The current emphasis is on that fundamental body unit the cell itself, and although detailed knowledge of intracellular processes and activities is being built up, the cell does not yield its secrets easily. It appears that new discoveries are harder to obtain but this is really only because we are at the stage of producing a new subsoil of 'enabling science'. On perhaps a more practical level, as the developments of the last thirty-five years have proceeded, new animal testing procedures have also been developed in order to evaluate the chemical compounds produced in thousands by the chemist and clinical research has become more and more refined, and within the limits of the human state, more and more exact. The contribution that pharmacologists, toxicologists, pharmacists and clinicians have made and are making to the overall progress of drug development will be referred to in the various chapters which follow. At the moment it is sufficient to emphasise yet again the fully integrated nature of successful research and development.

3
Basic Scientific Characterisation

CHEMICAL

Where does it all start? As we have seen in the previous chapter, chemical identification of therapeutically useful substances commenced with their isolation from naturally occurring materials. Once the constituent chemicals in naturally occurring substances of *vegetable* origin had been separated (often a difficult task since they usually consist of complicated mixtures) they could then be individually identified. As this occurred in the wake of the burgeoning science of chemistry, it was not long in many instances before the individual constituents could be synthesised by different routes rather than relying on extraction processes for a suitable supply.

Modification of Natural Effector Substances

Another source of therapeutic leads arose following the advent of biological research in the late nineteenth and early twentieth centuries. Naturally occurring substances within the *animal* body which produced pharmacological effects were identified chemically and copied. As we have seen, when chemical expertise had been developed, the multiplicity of compounds for the treatment of, for instance, hypertension became possible as the basic pharmacological mediators were chemically modified in various ways. This same principle was followed through perhaps less rigidly with the development of the non-steroidal anti-inflammatory agents and other therapeutic substances. Later on, with the identification and quantification of activity, new chemical leads are created and a 'mushrooming' effect occurs with compounds which have dissimilar structures from the root compound being made which possess activity in various organs and body systems.

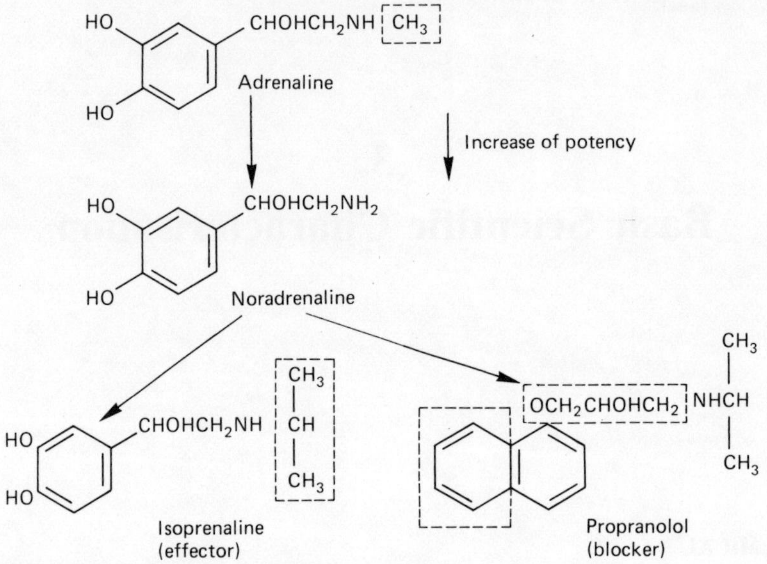

Figure 11   Once the natural substances adrenaline and noradrenaline (which lacks part of the adrenaline structure) had been identified, the way was clear for the synthesis of more precisely acting effector ('mimicking') substances such as isoprenaline and blocking compounds – e.g. propranolol. Blocking compounds have wide utility in medicine, cutting out the effects of noradrenaline which might be harmful or inappropriate.

'Molecular Roulette'

A third method of creating major leads occurred as pharmaceutical science itself advanced after World War II. Since chemists could turn out chemical compounds with great precision and speed, it became essential to test them in a battery of normal and abnormal physiological situations in order to identify their propensity to alter function and to attempt to predict their utility in man. Many compounds have been rapidly examined under this type of regime (which virtually all research laboratories use) and vast numbers have been rejected for either absence of effect, inappropriate effects or overt toxicity. However, many substances with useful properties have been discovered by this rather arbitrary methodology which is briefly described below.

Let us assume then that a scientist has conceived in his mind's eye a structure which he believes might be therapeutically useful. The concept will be built on his knowledge and experience but may have a significant component of serendipity. The next step is to make that compound. It may be easy or difficult. Assuming that a small quantity has been made, the chemist will now proceed to prepare it in a pure form, and to check that what he thinks he has made is actually what exists. At this stage it will be characterised using various simple and sophisticated analytical techniques.

Early Manufacture and Animal Testing

Before the research investigation for therapeutic utility can be moved forward the next stage must be to make an adequate quantity for initial pharmacological testing, since if the compound is without any useful effect or is overtly toxic there is no point in proceeding further. To maximise scarce resources the object is to answer this fundamental question as soon as possible. When prepared in adequate amount, the chemical in a pure form will be administered to a few experimental animals and the effects in these animals carefully observed (see next section).

It is possible even at this very early stage to get a rough idea of the effects exhibited by the compound and its relative potency. Depending upon the effects observed, when in a small number of animals 50% exhibit an effect, a crude arithmetical measure of the effective dose (ED 50) is established. Similarly, that dose which when administered to a group of rodents kills 50% of them is designated the lethal dose (LD 50). These are two very early crude estimates of the effective and toxic levels of the compound. Obviously ideally the two values should be widely separated. Recently there has been much examination of the relevance of this LD 50 test since many argue it uses animals for very little actual gain in knowledge. It is interesting to note in this context that Thalidomide has an enormously high LD 50 which means that great amounts can be given to animals without producing any serious toxicity. As later events showed this measurement bears no relationship to the compounds' real toxicological spectrum, that is the type of noxious effects to be observed in man (see later).

Pilot Batch Manufacture

Assuming all looks good at this initial stage, before any further pharmacological and toxicological work can be carried out a further supply of the new chemical to an acceptable and constant degree of purity must be assured, since all of the later research will be founded upon this fact. It is clearly desirable to have all animal and human work performed using identical material. A guaranteed supply of this is essential to the smooth running of any subsequent research and development programme.

This supply will probably be the pilot batch and about this time formulation studies (see later) will start. Thereafter pharmaceutical chemists will be occupied identifying in detail the synthesis whereby the original quantities were prepared and continually scaling up production to provide adequate quantities for formal pharmacological and toxicological evaluation. The route of the original synthesis must therefore be worked out in detail and accurately described.

The whole process of chemical production which follows is one of precise checks and controls. It commences with the establishment of the specifications of the starting materials which are accurately characterised in terms of appearance, melting point, purity, etc. As the synthetic route to produce the final chemical is followed through, the yield of product at each stage is carefully monitored. Obviously, in any chemical process the quantity of product will not be directly equivalent to the quantities of starting material since unwanted side reactions may occur together with consequent losses from this and other sources. The quality of the intermediates must be checked as the synthetic route proceeds and they are specifically investigated in terms of their appearance, melting point, etc. It follows naturally from this that the more complex the synthesis the more costly is the ultimate pure chemical.

Establishment of Final Specification

Eventually the final purification stage is reached and inevitably some small degree of impurity will be present although most pharmaceutical substances nowadays are prepared to extremely high standards of purity even when produced in batches of many tonnes. Incidentally, a batch is that quantity manufactured or prepared as one complete 'run' of the process or procedure. Depending on the dose level of the new product candidate, work will already be proceeding on the problems of 'scale-up' (this is chemical process development). As scale-up occurs, the impurity pattern will probably be the same as with smaller batches but it may not be. Impurities can arise not only from the starting materials (which may be different in large-scale manufacture) but also from the synthetic process itself. The methods for detection, identification and evaluation of any impurities in the final product will all need to be described precisely.

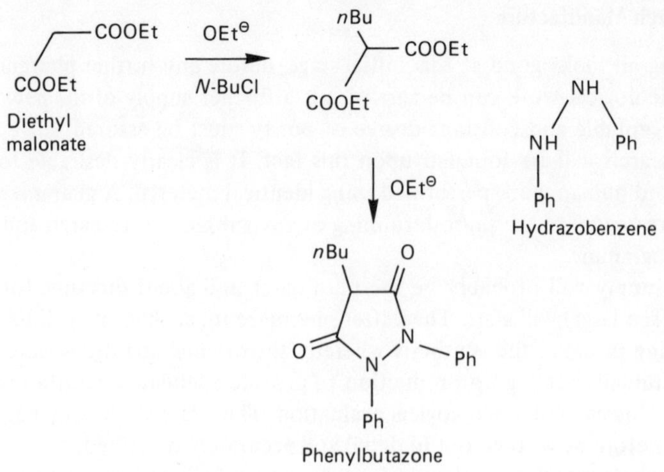

Figure 12   A simple short synthesis which employs readily available, cheap materials and which gives a good yield.

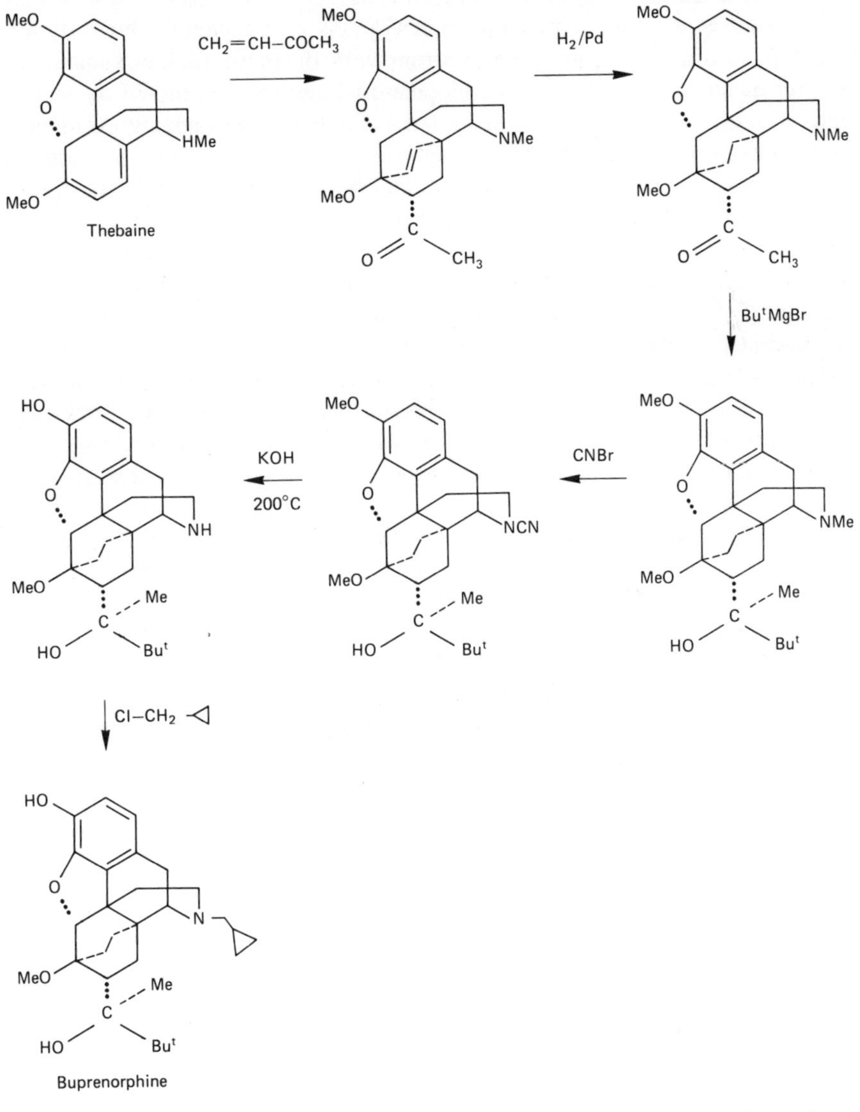

Figure 13 An example of an intermediate-length synthesis to produce the analgesic bupre-
norphine. Because the chemistry is complicated, the final product is expensive to produce.

This procedure, designed to assure adequate quantities of acceptably pure chemical, will occupy many months and will involve many people in much painstaking work.

The synthesis itself may need modification as it is scaled up since the problems which arise as a result of preparing a few grams in a chemical laboratory are likely to be dissimilar from those occurring with the preparation of kilogram or greater quantities in a chemical development laboratory, and these may be different again from the problems encountered in preparing vast quantities (tonnes) of the chemical in huge industrial complexes especially built and commissioned for the purpose. However, notwithstanding the scale of production the appropriate checks must be present throughout. As a result of this it may become apparent that the original synthesis cannot be appropriately scaled up but work in other areas (pharmacology, toxicology and perhaps chemical) has by this time become extensive. The problem then is to devise a new synthesis which can be appropriately scaled up and which will produce material to the already established specification for the final product since all of the other work will have been done using chemicals with this specification. If this cannot be achieved there may be a problem with comparability of the results and certain of the investigations may have to be repeated. Alternatively, a synthesis may be changed because a cheaper route has been discovered.

The final objective here and the hoped-for end result is to be able to describe precisely the method of manufacture of the finished product, whether it is a solid or a liquid, to be absolutely sure that it is of the stated degree of purity and that the impurity profile is known, predictable and constant between very narrow limits.

This final product characterisation will consist of a description of the physical form, colour, odour and other physical characteristics of the compound and its:

- Structural formula
- Molecular formula
- Molecular weight
- Solubility in various substances
- Infra-red absorption spectrum
- Ultra-violet absorption spectrum
- Thin-layer chromatography
- Ash residue
- Weight loss on drying
- pH of suspension/solution
- Assay
- Solvent content

In addition to the above, information on the thermal characteristics, polymorphism, pK_a value, solubility and isomerism may be necessary. The importance of the contribution of the skilled analyst using very sophisticated modern tech-

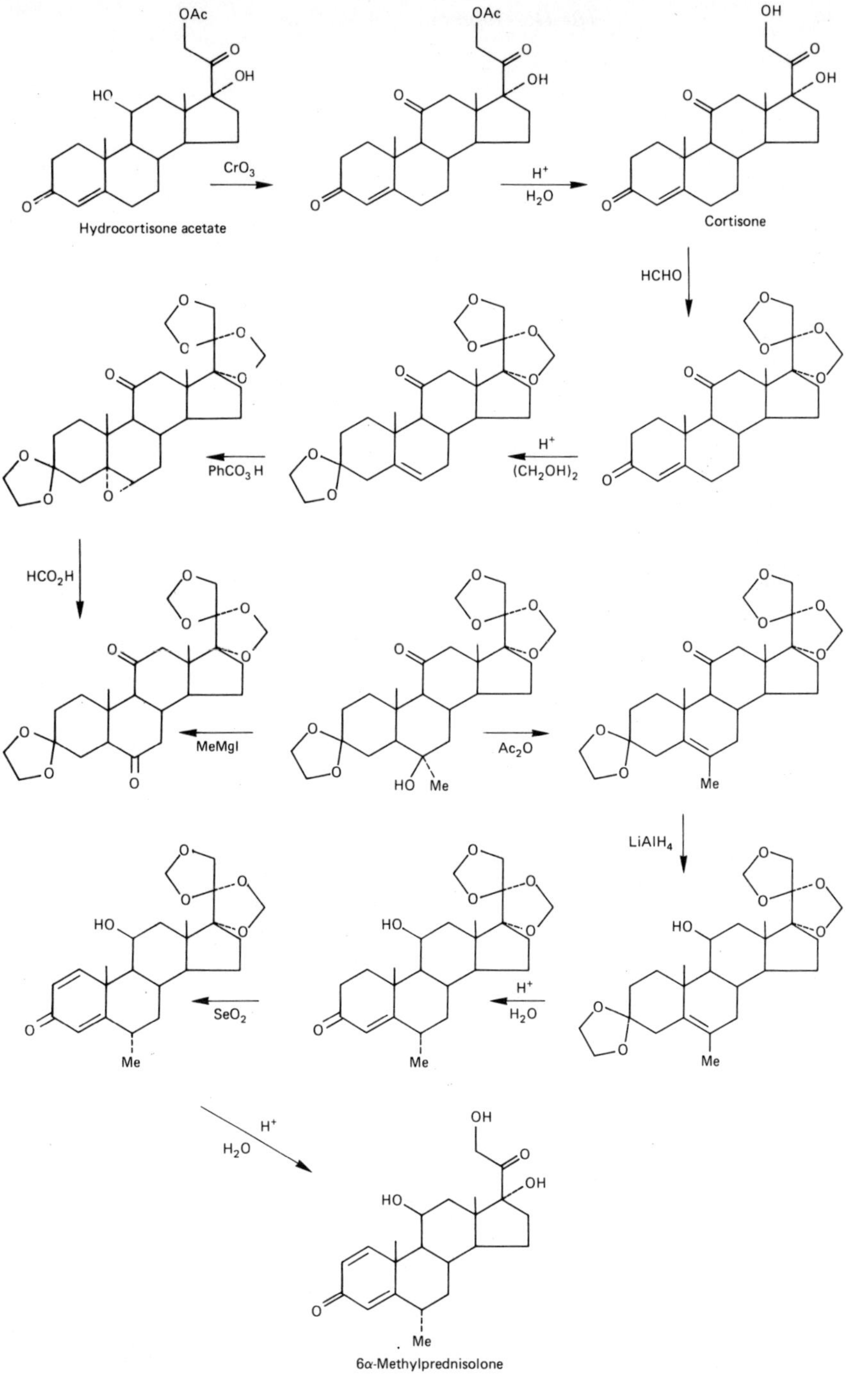

Figure 14 Examples of long complicated synthesis where, because of low yields of intermediate compounds together with reagent and labour costs, the cost of the final product is many times higher than that of the starting materials.

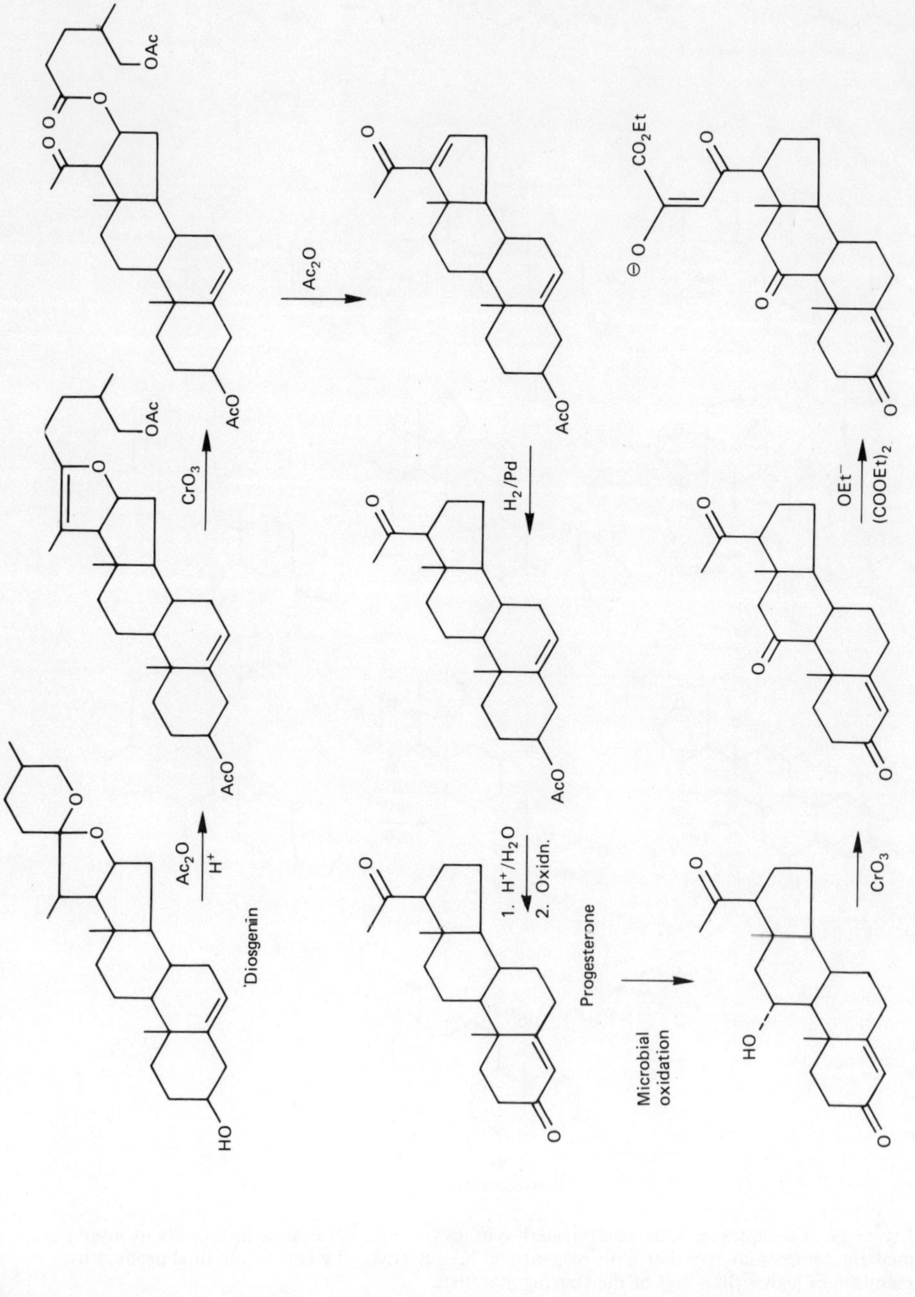

Figure 14 (continued)

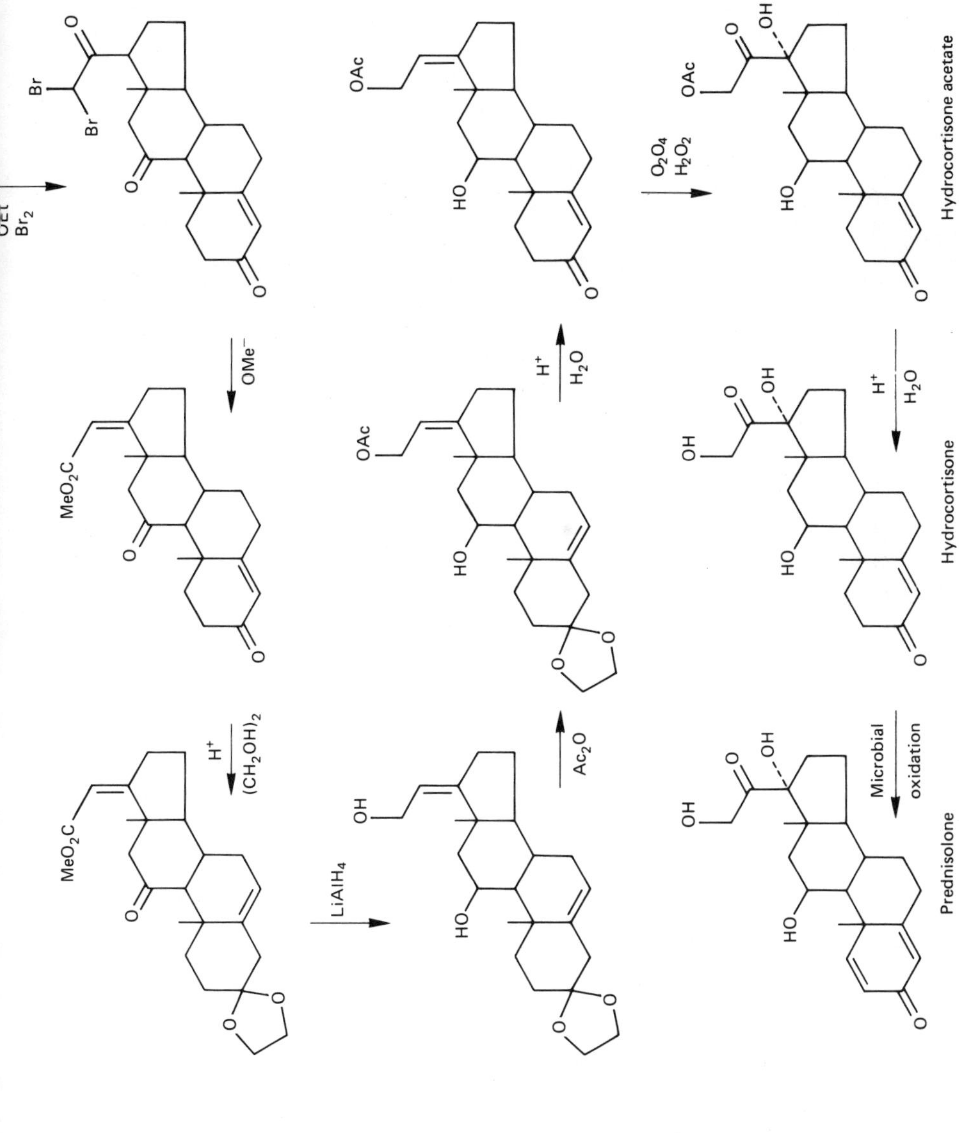

Figure 14 (continued)

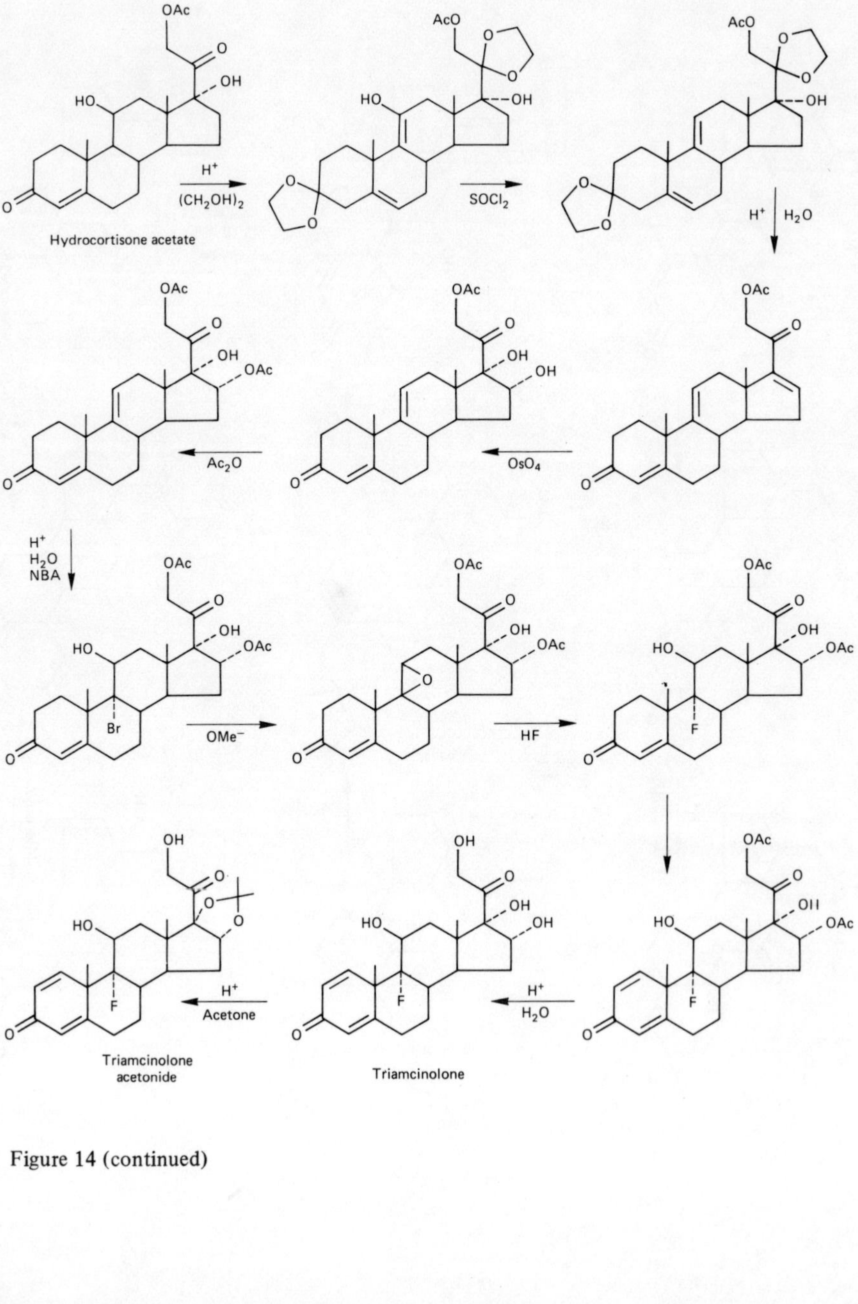

Figure 14 (continued)

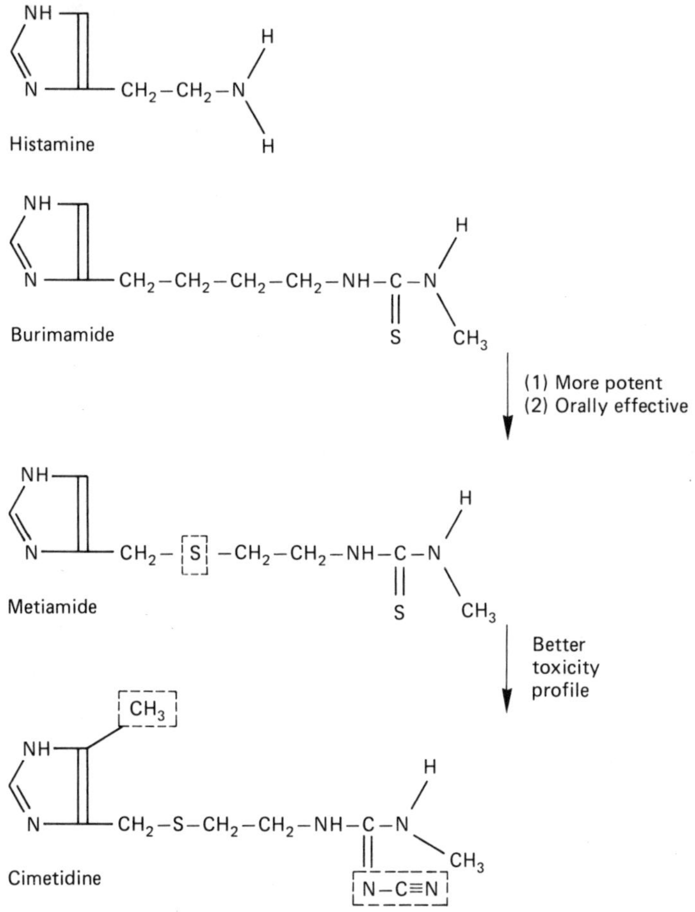

NH

N — CH$_2$—CH$_2$—N(H)(H)

Histamine

NH

N — CH$_2$—CH$_2$—CH$_2$—CH$_2$—NH—C—N(H)(CH$_3$)
‖
S

Burimamide

(1) More potent
(2) Orally effective

NH

N — CH$_2$— [S] —CH$_2$—CH$_2$—NH—C—N(H)(CH$_3$)
‖
S

Metiamide

Better
toxicity
profile

[CH$_3$]

NH

N — CH$_2$—S—CH$_2$—CH$_2$—NH—C—N(H)(CH$_3$)
‖
[N—C≡N]

Cimetidine

Figure 15 Molecular development of cimetidine to safely and effectively block the actions of the natural substance histamine.

niques cannot be understated or underestimated since all of this long and complicated process (together with some later studies) is designed to assure *quality*.

In summary, new medicines can arise by a number of different routes. Ideally perhaps a new drug will originate as a rational design based upon previous knowledge of what certain chemical groupings will do in the animal body. As an extension of this, chemical modification of an existing synthetic drug or a therapeutically proven natural substance, or indeed incorporation of a pharmacologically active grouping (pharmacophore) into a novel substrate, may all produce a viable new lead. Using a serendipitous approach on the other hand, the new medicine could originate through the prolific production of novel chemicals which are then screened for biological activity. The actual derivation of the new

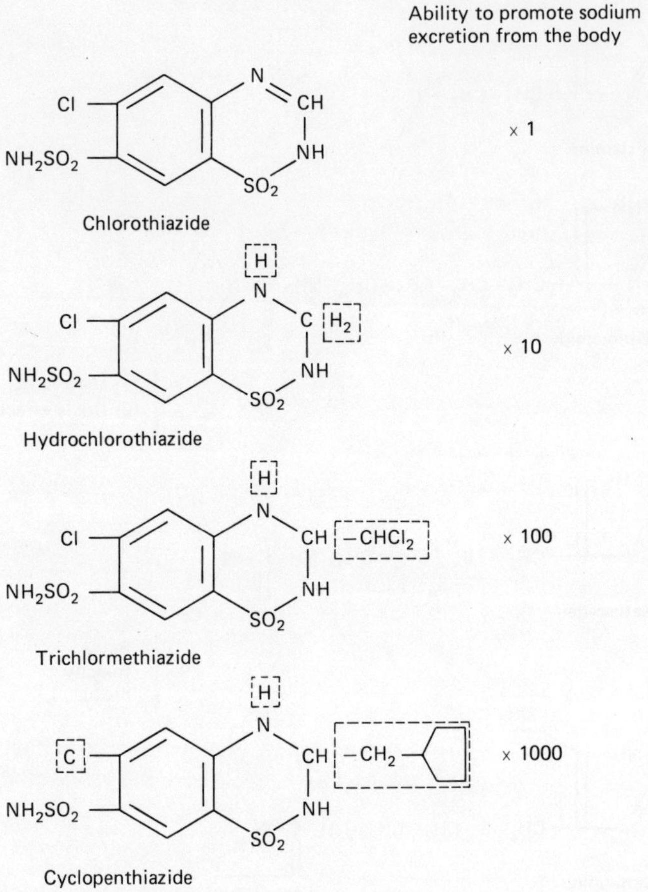

Figure 16   An example of so-called 'molecular roulette', where the alteration of a molecule in particular ways can enhance a specific therapeutic effect. However, the position of the substitution and the type of group employed can produce significant differences in the toxicity profile.

lead will depend upon the mixture of skills available to a pharmaceutical company, the philosophy of its scientists, its cash resources and the imagination and courage of its leadership.

BIOLOGICAL

In practice, biological characterisation, safety evaluation and proof of efficacy are closely intertwined and therefore both this and following sections should be read with this constantly in mind. But, because so much work takes place coincidentally it is extremely difficult, and perhaps in the long run not very helpful, to break it down artificially. By the same token, in the previous section the progress of a chemical substance from an idea to the production possibly of tonne quantities has been outlined. It should however be re-emphasised that this process takes months or even years to complete. In order to ensure a constant supply of suitable material for all of the subsequent animal and human investigations however, it must interlock accurately with them at all stages.

Now that the scientist has devised a chemical substance which is supposed to have utility in a certain human disease state, the next stage of development is devoted either to the qualitative proving or disproving of this hypothesis. If it is indeed true the pharmacologist will also go on not only to quantify the main effect but also to identify and quantify the secondary effects of the compound.

Advances in Experimental Methods

Whereas in the early days of pharmacological investigation experiments consisted, for example, of injecting substances into animals and either observing gross alterations in their behaviour or trying to record various changes using Heath Robinsonian arrangements recording on to smoked drums, the whole basis of the science has changed dramatically in recent years. Nowadays methods of investigation of drug effects and particularly their recording have become so refined that the effects of substances down to nanogram (10^{-9}) and even picogram (10^{-12}) quantities can be detected. These effects, accurately recorded by electronic and other means, can be monitored over very tiny units of time (milliseconds). However, the above levels of precision and accuracy are something which are arrived at during the course of a research and development programme. Recordings start simply and build up to greater and greater degrees of delicacy. Indeed this is the watchword of the whole drug development process – experiments are simple and straightforward at first, becoming more refined and complicated as the investigation proceeds. However, even in the initial stages, techniques have advanced significantly since the days of the smoked drum. They are considerably less open to error and misinterpretation. This is obviously important in order to secure a sound foundation for the ensuing investigations.

Pharmacology in Normal Animals

The new drug candidate is first administered both by mouth and by injection (parenterally) to healthy anaesthetised animals, usually mice or other small rodents (but also dogs, cats, guinea pigs, rabbits and certain primates may be employed at different stages), and the effects observed. These can be separated into primary and secondary effects. Of particular interest are investigations into the effects of the new compound on the dynamics of the cardiovascular system, its influence on the central nervous system and the performance of respiratory studies. By comparing the degree of effect between oral and intra-

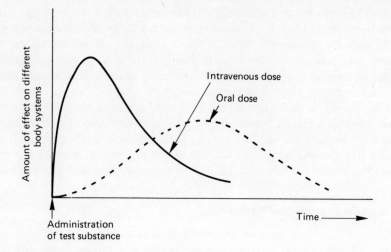

Figure 17   The speed of onset, the degree and the time for return to baseline levels can be assessed using, say, intravenous and oral dosing and carefully observing effects on heart rate, respiratory rate, etc.

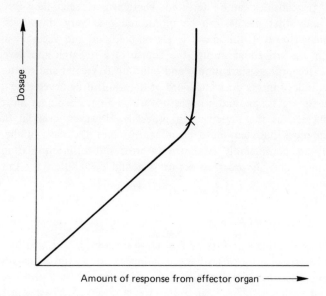

Figure 18   Increasing the dose of a pharmacologically active substance will produce increasing responses from the effector organ up to a certain point when response is maximal. This point is indicated by a cross on the diagram and increasing the dosage beyond this is valueless, since it produces no further increment in effect but may well increase the risk of toxicity.

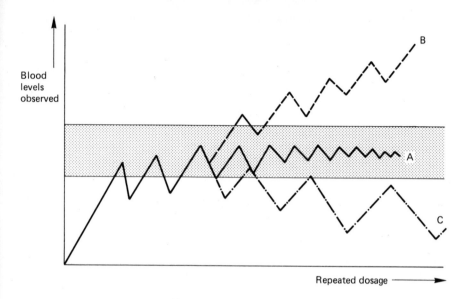

Figure 19 Effects of repeated dosage. The shaded area represents the ideal therapeutic range of the drug. The ideal state is shown by A, where after a number of doses a steady state of input versus output (dosage versus excretion and metabolism) occurs. In B, if dosage is excessive or excretion and metabolism cannot cope even with normal dosage, accumulation of the drug in the body may occur, with probable toxic effects. In C, however, if dosage is inadequate or metabolism and excretion very effective, the drug will be therapeutically inefficient.

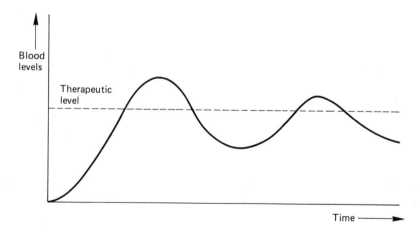

Figure 20 Showing the effect of storage of a medicine in, say, body fat. The drug may emerge later to exert a therapeutic effect. Clearly this would be a disadvantage with a hypnotic, since it could produce somnolence at an inappropriate time.

venous dosing, an early view can be obtained of the capability of the animals to absorb the compound effectively via the alimentary tract.

Some compounds are so rapidly and effectively destroyed, either by gastric acid or other intestinal juices or indeed by enzyme systems located within the gut wall, that their later utility as therapeutic agents may be significantly impaired. However, it may be possible by applying modern chemical and formulation knowledge to overcome such a problem (as in the case of penicillin).

Having administered single doses to healthy animals and observed the effects, the next step is to ascertain the effect of dosage increments. The new compound may exhibit dose response curves which are regular and linear, but they may not be. After this early stage the pattern of dose response will be investigated further both in animals and man. In addition the effect of multiple dosing (over hours and days) will need to be studied. Information from these studies will give pointers to the likelihood or not of accumulation of the agent which may be matched with signs of toxicity. Already then, knowledge about the new compound is starting to build up, but essentially the studies so far have been performed in normal animals.

Pharmacology in Disease Models

Logically we must now try to obtain a view of the new compound's utility in the abnormal (disease) state we wish to affect. Leading on from the general investigation in normal animals, virtually all laboratories nowadays subject the new chemical to a whole series of specialised animal tests in order to establish its effects more precisely (both primary and secondary) in relation to various body systems which are in an abnormal or diseased state. Because animals do not necessarily exhibit the same diseases or conditions which can afflict humanity, a great amount of work has been done over the years in order to obtain reliable and reproducible animal models of conditions mimicking human disease states. As might be expected, some of these are more successfully predictive than others.

Again the effects are studied in terms of single and multiple doses and the aim is to establish a view of the pattern and type of dose response. Many of these models are skilfully devised and have themselves been studied minutely over long periods of time. Examples are numerous and include artificially induced arthritis (e.g. carragenin paw oedema, adjuvant arthritis) and artificially induced hypertension in rats (various operative and biochemical procedures). In fact test systems exist for virtually every human disease state. Their basic purpose is to establish a degree of predictability regarding the profile of the new drug candidate which with reasonable certainty might be applied to the human condition. Of course these test procedures can exhibit from time to time false positives and false negatives, but since no one test is used in isolation, the chances of a serious mistake in establishing the profile are much diminished. It is not the purpose of this book to describe the great variety of these tests and procedures

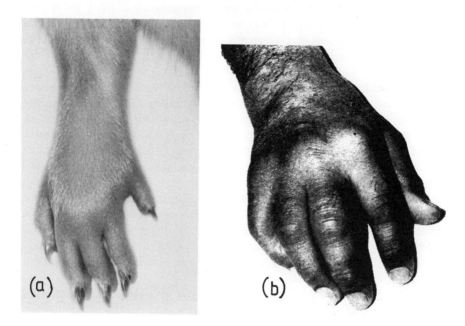

Figure 21 The similarity between artificially induced rat and human (rheumatoid) arthritis can be seen.

in detail. Suffice it to say that pharmaceutical science has devised and improved upon its own methods of establishing a compounds profile in a whole spectrum of different animal species in a great variety of different test procedures which mimic human conditions. It should also be mentioned that during all of these procedures the skilled researcher is cognisant of the welfare of the animals he uses in his experiments and of course is duly licensed to do such work by the appropriate body such as the Home Office.

The Spectrum of Investigation

The importance of a wide range of investigations cannot be over-emphasised, particularly with regard to the establishment of not only primary effects but also the agent's secondary actions. For instance, in animal studies investigating very active and ostensibly very useful anti-inflammatory agents (as indicated for instance by the carragenin paw oedema and other appropriate tests), it might be shown that they adversely affect the gastric lining and might also cause unwanted retention of salt and water. Alternatively, as a plus point they might in addition have the property of being significantly antipyretic. How compounds will actually fair in development will naturally depend on the qualitative and quantitative differences between these plus and minus parameters. Every active compound by virtue of its very activity will have some drawbacks, but it is very much a question of degree even at this early stage and all future work will be directed towards assessing the balance between the desired and unwanted effects.

After healthy animals and artificially induced disease models, isolated organs or tissues may be useful adjuncts in further investigating the compound's profile. Indeed biochemical experiments *in vitro* may also contribute significant segments of knowledge. These latter two approaches often provide important confirmatory evidence with regard to the more detailed characteristics of the compound's activity at the cellular or sub-cellular level. The basic reason for all tests and procedures is to gain *predictability* of the likely effects of the compound when it is administered to man. In many instances correlation is good, but in others it is less so. Over the years much time and effort has been devoted by many scientists to increasing the quality of this predictability. New tests are continually being devised with the continuing aim of simplicity, reliability, reproducibility and accuracy of correlation to the pathophysiology of the disease process it is desired to abolish or combat.

As already mentioned, scientists engaged in this work are naturally concerned about the welfare of the animals involved. They spend significant amounts of time refining methodologies so that, wherever possible, animal systems can be phased out by substituting various biochemical and cell-culture techniques. This, if successful, would have a number of advantages, not the least of which would be an increase in the likelihood of predictability because it would eliminate variations in response between individual animals. Therefore if this were possible on a wider scale, since it is reasonable to assume that the test system would have to fulfil many or all of the criteria listed above (clear scientific advantage), it would additionally be much cheaper. In times of rising costs, such a clear economic advantage could not fail to be attractive. Nowadays this aspect of development work is in its infancy but progress is continually being made.

Early Bioavailability Studies

So far we have accumulated knowledge of the pharmacodynamic profile of the new drug in both normal and abnormal animals (i.e. those with an approximation of the human disease state). That is, how much given over what period of time, does what? Assuming nothing grossly untoward has been identified so far we are now in a position to investigate in much more detail the pharmacokinetics of the compound, in other words how it is absorbed and handled by the body. First in this is the absorption of the drug. Is it effectively absorbed by mouth or not? Since medicines are most conveniently taken by mouth either as tablets, powders or suspensions, the capacity for effective oral absorption is clearly important. Known amounts are therefore given to animals, and by blood sampling over time the pattern of absorption and the quantities of the compound absorbed are measured.

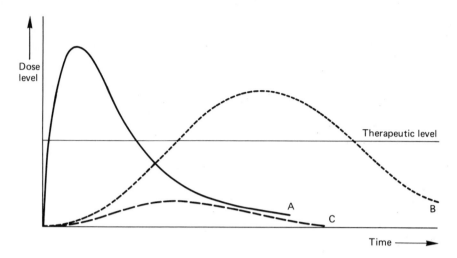

Figure 22 Showing how, with intravenous dosing, all the dose enters the body over a short timescale. However, with oral dosage a longer time is needed to achieve therapeutic levels, which may persist for longer. Curve C indicates an 'absorption failure' with a rectal suppository which never achieves a therapeutic level.

Similar measurements would be made if it was anticipated that the new compound would be given as a suppository or was intended for cutaneous application, or indeed for intramuscular injection. The speed of absorption is significant since the level to which the concentration in the blood rises over time may have an important bearing on its pharmacological effect. This is particularly true of compounds intended to be given by both intravenous and intramuscular injection. The quantity available to the body following an injection may determine the efficacy or harmfulness of the substance. Assuming that after an intravenous injection all of the substance is available to exert a pharmacological effect, the speed of the injection which will govern the concentration of the drug in the body may well be critical in determining the observed effects. A ready example is that of morphine which if given slowly has certain analgesic and other central nervous system effects, but if given very rapidly as a 'bolus' could kill a morphine-naïve recipient.

Half-life Studies

Where drugs are intended to be given as eye or ear drops their capacity to produce pharmacological effects must also be carefully worked out. In all of these studies the object will be to obtain a value for the mean absorption half-life, that is, what is the unit of time in which half of the administered dose is fully and effectively absorbed? The effectiveness of absorption of the compound will also be checked at this time by administering a known amount of

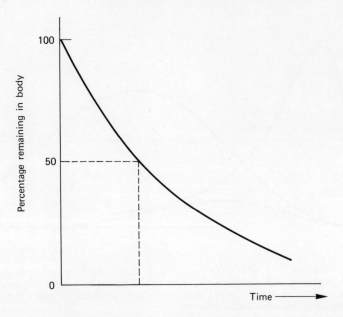

Figure 23 The half-life of a compound is that time when half of an administered dose is present in the body. This will vary with the route of administration, since with an intra-venous dose all will enter the body in a short period of time. With an oral dose, however, not all may be absorbed.

radio-labelled compound (depending upon the compound's characteristics — labelled with carbon 14 or other radioactive isotope) both orally and intra-venously. These studies are normally performed in dogs, rats and monkeys and the end result of these investigations will be to confirm what are the likely peak plasma levels following (initially) single doses of varying amounts.

Distribution

Once absorbed within the body, the distribution of the compound is clearly important. Whether the compound passes the blood–brain barrier or, indeed, whether there is untoward accumulation in one or more tissues or body sites, could well be significant in later development. It may be a property which is highly desirable. On the other hand it could be singularly inappropriate and give rise to deleterious effects such as to prejudice seriously later development of the compound. These effects can be checked in two major ways. Firstly, tissue samples can be taken and chemically analysed to establish the quantity of the compound contained in them. Secondly, this can also be done in a more refined manner by administering the compound in a radioactive form to small animals. After suitable time intervals the animals are killed and the whole-animal bodies frozen. Using a microtome, frozen sections of the whole animals are cut

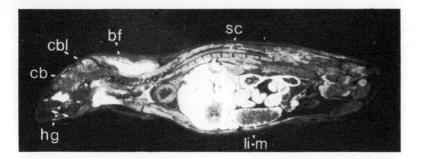

1h

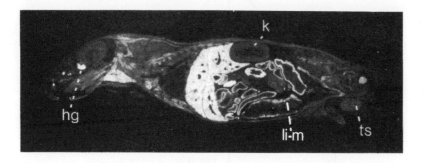

6h

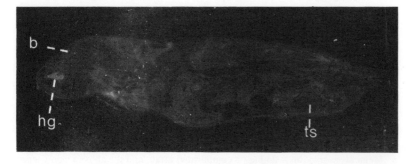

72h

Figure 24 Whole-body autoradiograms of a male mouse. After 1 h the radioactive drug is concentrated widely throughout the animal's body (white appearance). After 6 h only the liver and a few other organs show up white, indicating that most of the drug has been eliminated. This is confirmed by the picture at 72 h, which shows practically no residual radioactivity.

and placed on an x-ray plate. These thin tissue slices, by virtue of the radio-activity contained in them, will affect the x-ray plate to produce auto-radio-graphs. For obvious reasons small mammals are the most suitable for these investigations. When the x-ray plates are developed it enables the investigator to identify immediately whether any organ is a site of selective uptake or if there is a specific pattern of distribution. This information can also be plotted over time since a series of animals can be sacrificed at different time intervals after dosing.

Metabolism

Having been absorbed and distributed around the body (usually by the blood vessels) the compound will be subjected to various degrees and types of body

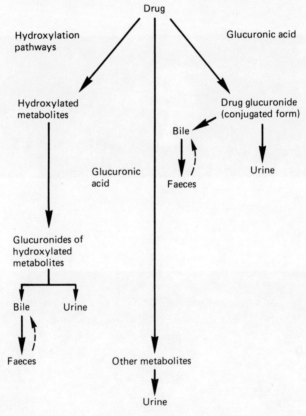

Figure 25   Metabolism may be a simple or complicated affair, and the above schema represents only a few such possibilities. However, the object is either to excrete the drug unchanged or to change (biotransform) it in some way. This will allow it to be eliminated either via the urine or the bile (and then into the faeces) or a combination of both. The body may be frustrated or aided in its designs by either strong or weak plasma protein binding of a drug, interactions with other drugs, circulation between the gut and the liver (enterohepatic circulation) or irregular or incomplete elimination by the kidney.

metabolism. Of course a certain amount of it may have been extensively metabolised before absorption has taken place (metabolised in the enzyme systems of the gut wall). At the further end of the scale, it may have been neither metabolised nor absorbed by the gut wall and may be excreted in the faeces unchanged. Clearly this would be a gross disadvantage for a cardiovascular drug since it would mean the only way of making it bio-available would be by intramuscular or intravenous injection. However, if it were intended as a treatment for diarrhoea or to kill intestinal worms, this property would be clearly advantageous since it would enable the drug candidate to be targeted where required. If it were not absorbed the likelihood of adverse or inappropriate effects elsewhere in the body would be either much diminished or eliminated. However, most compounds are metabolised to some degree and metabolism by the liver and kidneys is usually by well-recognised paths. Sometimes the absorbed drug candidate is inactive but is converted by a process of metabolism to an active compound. In this instance the parent compound is said to be a *pro-drug* and it will depend for its pharmacological activity on the host's processes of metabolism. The question of timescale of the metabolism is in this instance extremely important. Alternatively, the drug may be metabolised to a more toxic compound than the original agent or indeed a metabolite may have target organ toxicity. Again compounds metabolised by the liver and excreted into the bile can be the subject of a re-uptake between the gut and the liver as the excreted compound is reabsorbed (enterohepatic recycling). Furthermore there may be auto-induction (increase) of metabolism of the compound by its effects on hepatic enzymes.

Interactions

Often the drug is designed to be taken in conditions where other already established medicaments are commonly co-administered. Therefore the question of absorption interactions will become important. There may also be heteroinduction of the metabolism of the new compound by other agents. Of course, chemical compounds are protein bound (i.e. attached to plasma proteins) to varying degrees. Affinity for plasma proteins varies between compounds. Some compounds displace others, and the compound's physical behaviour in this respect will have a bearing on the pharmacological action and the distribution achieved together with its metabolism and elimination (since only the unbound fraction is available for these activities and processes).

Excretion

Finally, the pattern of excretion from the animal body must be investigated. We have already seen that some compounds may be excreted via the bile into the gut only to be the subject of re-uptake. Other compounds may be excreted via the kidneys. The majority of compounds are eliminated from the body by various combinations of these two major routes (liver, kidneys) although they can also be eliminated by other routes (skin, sweat, tears).

The time at which all of the introduced compound has been removed from the body is important since if removal is not efficient or occurs over a very long timescale, accumulation may result. Persistence in the body, if it occurs, will be extensively investigated because of its highly important bearing on the establishment of a dosage regime and its relationship to toxicity (see later).

All of the above investigations will be initially performed using single doses, but will rapidly proceed to multiple dose investigations. They are designed to give adjunctive information on how much of the new drug needs to be given to produce the desired effect, and how frequently. The metabolism studies are important as a foundation for later work and because these investigations are done in a variety of animals, different routes of metabolism will be identified in different species. Of course, in the later investigations it will be important to perform the toxicity evaluation in a species which handles the compound by the same routes as man (see later). In all of these studies the importance of analytical capability is clearly apparent. Virtually all of the work is founded on accurate and effective methods of detection of the parent compound and its metabolites in body fluids. Whereas the actual levels of the compound in blood may or may not be important in determining degree of therapeutic effect (see later), they can be significant in arriving at estimates of the compound's behaviour in the animal body. The constant need for high analytical skill and capability cannot be overstressed. Many research and development programmes have been seriously delayed through its paucity.

Biological characterisation will therefore have established in animals some answers to questions such as how much needs to be given to do what, how long do the effects last and how long do they take to wear off, and do they leave any deleterious effects in their wake. The answers to these (pharmacological) questions will also be accompanied by information on the capability of the body to absorb the compound (from the gut or an injection site), distribute it, metabolise it and excrete it by whatever route. These latter studies will also provide a logical foundation for the ensuing safety evaluation exercise.

4

Safety Evaluation (Animal Studies)

By this stage of the investigation quite a considerable amount of work has already been done in relation to the new drug candidate. We have an early view that it can be made by a feasible chemical route and that the necessary raw materials are available to a requisite standard of purity. We know also that the new compound has distinct effects in normal and abnormal intact animals and also in various isolated tissue and biochemical preparations. What we do not yet know is how safe it is or alternatively how toxic it might be following chronic administration to either animals or man.

An early view of acute toxicity has already been obtained using the LD 50 test. This is done by different routes of administration (oral, intraperitoneal and intravenous — this latter of course gives absolute assurance that the quantity administered has entered the animal body). The test may be performed using rats, mice or guinea pigs and only very occasionally are other species used. It must of necessity (in the absence of any other information) be done on a trial and error basis. Using mice, groups of 20 animals (10 females and 10 males) are dosed and the death rate observed. There may be a differential lethality between the sexes. After a number of experiments the LD 50 is established. It may be approximately $\times 70$-$\times 100$ more than the prospective human dose, it may be only $\times 2$ or $\times 3$. Whatever the level is it will give a guide to the compound's potential for mischief. This will not be an absolute since it is widely known that the correlation between animal and human toxicity is not altogether accurate and predictive.

TOXICOLOGICAL TESTING AND IMPORTANCE OF CONTROL GROUPS

Using the information gained in the dose response work performed by the pharmacologists and described above, the toxicologist will now devise a short-term (7-day) toxicity test. This is usually done in mice and rats. Three dose levels will be selected where the lowest dose will be about two to five times the prospective human dose (calculated pro rata on a weight for weight basis) and predicted on the basis of the pharmacological experiments already performed. The top dose will be a multiple of the lowest dose, and again using the LD 50, information will be designed to produce overt toxicity and will probably be lethal to some of the animals. The middle dose is pitched at that level logarithmically between the lowest and highest dose. To ensure scientific validity a control group of animals is included which will be dosed with the vehicle(s) which the drug candidate has been mixed with (or, the formulation minus the drug). The animals are usually given the test substance on a once-a-day basis and on every day the test is in operation. The level and quantity of toxic effects will determine whether it is decided to proceed to testing in humans and also the dosage regime to be tried.

Over the years there have been many schemata for toxicity testing all of which are designed to determine the limits of risk with regard to human administration. It used to be accepted practice that after the 7-day experiment the toxicologist proceeded to 14-day and longer tests. Nowadays the tendency is to start a 3-month toxicity study using, for example, rats and dogs with provision to do a 'read out' at 28 days without disturbing the longer study. This is a decision which has to be taken at the outset because it requires more animals to be started in the study than would have been the case with a straightforward 3-months experiment.

Leading on from the 3-month study, when this is complete and the animals have been killed and subjected to post-mortem examination, a detailed report giving the procedure itself, the methods for monitoring the study and the outcome is written.

Since this is a longer-term experiment than the 7-day study mentioned above, it is possible that different toxic effects may have shown themselves. Should this be the case the matter has to be considered in detail with regard to the particular nature of the toxic effect together with the timescale and dose at which it became apparent. Such a finding may have an important bearing on the drug candidate's future and will depend upon the nature and timescale of the condition it is designed to treat.

LONGER-TERM ANIMAL STUDIES

If all looks good at the 3-month toxicity report stage it will be considered appropriate to move to a full 12-month study using rats, dogs and occasionally monkeys. Using knowledge gained in previous experiments, three dosage levels will again be selected together with a control group. As with earlier studies, steps will be taken to ensure that the animals are appropriately dosed with the test substance to ensure that they receive the drug-substance every day the test is running and that it is present in their bodies for a large part of every 24 hours. This is usually achieved by grinding up the substance to a degree of fineness where it can be effectively mixed with the animals' food, or it can be given via the drinking water. It can even be given directly to animals via a pipette or syringe (gavage). At all times during the conduct of the study the animals are closely observed and monitored. Various blood samples will be taken and analysed. Any animal showing signs of suffering is removed from the study and humanely sacrificed. At the end of twelve months the remaining animals are also humanely sacrificed and full post-mortem examination is carried out. A large definitive report detailing all the findings is then written.

CARCINOGENICITY TESTING

Following the successful conclusion of the 12-month study described above, the next stage is to proceed to the full 24-month investigation in two species (usually rats and mice), which is known as *carcinogenicity testing*. The object of this study, which lasts for virtually the entire life-span of the experimental animals, is to gauge whether any potential carcinogenic risk exists. A great deal is now known about the incidence of tumours and other malignancies in rats and mice of different types and strains, and the excess incidence of any neoplasm can usually be appreciated. The groups of animals are now much larger but are still equally divided between the sexes and a control group is included as before. The animals are kept in excellent conditions and are examined regularly by skilled personnel. As with earlier toxicity experiments, animals which show signs of undue suffering during the course of the experiment are humanely sacrificed and the post-mortem findings are recorded. Post-mortems are also performed

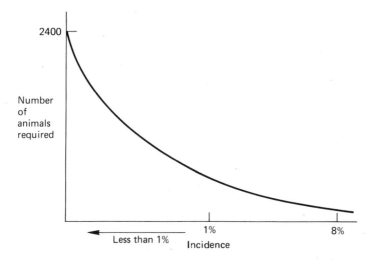

Figure 26 Showing the number of animals which would be needed in the experiment to be 90% sure of having at least one animal with a tumour, assuming *no* background incidence of that particular tumour. It can be seen that very large numbers of animals are required to be sure, particularly if the likely incidence is less than 1%.

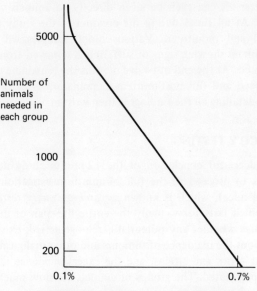

Figure 27   If the incidence of a certain type of tumour is only 0.1% in the control group, then the number of animals required to be 90% sure of detecting an *additional* likelihood of tumour in the tested group increases enormously.

on animals dying during the course of the study. At the end of the 2-year span all the animals are sacrificed and inspected post-mortem. All tumours or other malignant events are recorded and specimens are prepared from these and normal tissues. The whole exercise may take up to $3\frac{1}{2}$ years to complete. It is very expensive and consequently is not undertaken lightly. By the time a company has put a new compound into carcinogenicity testing it is a long way down the developmental road, well into clinical testing, and consequently has an expectation that the compound could eventually be marketed. The timing of such a test is therefore critical in terms of the optimum timescale of the drug's development, but has to be matched with the company's financial resources in relation to their competing projects.

FERTILITY STUDIES

However, before performing a carcinogenicity test there are other shorter-term experiments a company will carry out to be assured of safety in other directions. These will include fertility tests, where groups of rats (both males and females) are dosed with the new compound for a number of days prior to being mated. Following conception the female rats (dams) are allowed to proceed with pregnancy. Of these females, 50% are sacrificed the day before delivery is expected and their uteri are examined to determine whether any abnormal foetuses exist or indeed whether there are any obvious signs of resorption of the conceived foetuses (often a foetus which is damaged or blighted from whatever source does not continue to grow but dies in the uterus and is resorbed – the site of this resorption is detectable). The surviving 50% are allowed to deliver their 'pups' normally and go through lactation and weaning. The majority of the dams and pups (now mature) are then sacrificed and examined, but one pup from each litter is selected and mated with a non-related pup to produce another generation which is then sacrificed and examined as before. The point behind all of this procedure is to try and uncover agents which are toxic to the reproductive systems (both male and female) and which when administered to animals during the critical periods of their lives when their cells are rapidly dividing may give rise to untoward effects.

By the same token peri- and post-natal studies are done to elicit whether the new drug substance affects the abilities of both parents and offspring to behave normally and effectively at this stage in their existences.

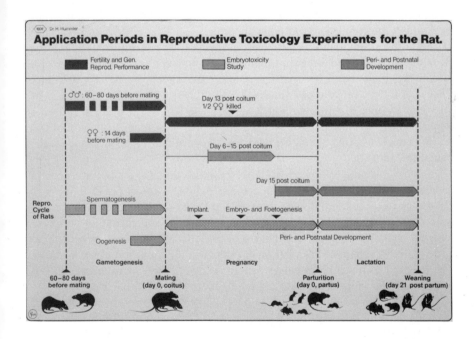

Figure 28 Showing how, geared to the reproductive cycle of the rat (shown below), the animals are dosed in order to expose them to the influence of the new drug at distinct phases of their lives. Thus the effects of the drug on sperm and egg formation, the implantation and future development of the embryo and fetus, the birth and weaning process and subsequent development can all be assessed.

TERATOLOGY

Usually having done the straightforward toxicity experiments extending over ever-lengthening periods of time together with the fertility and peri- and post-natal studies, a definitive teratology study is performed. This employs animals of two different species (rats and rabbits) and the aim is to dose them (again at three dosage levels) at a time when they are pregnant and the foetus is at a stage when its internal organs are forming (organogenesis). Thus the chemical insult (if in fact it is such) is applied at the most vulnerable time. Just before the normal time of delivery the dams are sacrificed and the foetuses are carefully examined with particular reference to the completeness or otherwise of their skeletons and internal organs, noting also whether everything is in its proper place. It is usual in these experiments to include a 'positive control'. This is a known teratogen — a substance well known for producing developmental defects.

All of the experiments so far described are a carefully ordered progression which seeks to build up knowledge on a new compound in order to enable decisions to be taken on its future at distinct stages, since the longer drug development proceeds the more costly it becomes. These experiments are also supplemented by various tests *in vitro* which attempt to identify whether or not a compound will produce mutations of living cells. Naturally, such studies are preliminary and adjunctive to the carcinogenicity tests described above.

As a rule, compounds which have a chemical or pharmacological relation to either a known or suspect carcinogen or mutagen, or a metabolite of a carcinogen or mutagen (or a co-carcinogen), are required to be so tested since they may affect cell division (mitosis). In addition, compounds which may be innocent as judged above but which are likely to be present or retained in the human body for long periods or used chronically (for more than six months) by humans (especially young people) have to be tested for their carcinogenic/ mutagenic potential.

As with toxicity testing, it is clearly essential that the studies are done in animal species exhibiting similar metabolic pathways for disposal of the new substance to those used in man. Therefore the necessity for dovetailing is easily seen. Enough toxicity testing must be done to permit administration to man in order to investigate human metabolism so that this information can be used to generate more complete information in animals so that in turn the new medicine can be given to humans for longer periods of time. It is a circus movement and requires careful judgement to act responsibly in an optimum timescale.

MUTAGENICITY STUDIES

These do not come in quite the same category as toxicity and carcinogenicity studies (above) in terms of requiring a degree of human feedback, but if the drug is related to a known mutagen or carcinogen (either chemically, biochemically or pharmacologically), or if in animal studies it is suspected that it may affect the reproductive system, depress bone marrow (another site of rapidly dividing cells) or exert a teratogenic effect, it must be tested. In fact various tests have now been developed which yield much valuable information. They employ bacteria (*Salmonella typhimurium*), yeasts and various mammalian cells. They can indicate liability to produce gene mutations, chromosomal damage (ruptures and anomalies) or whether DNA repair is adversely affected.

This chapter has described a whole battery of tests stemming from the acute and relatively unsophisticated LD 50 down to the detailed 12-month toxicity, fertility and teratology tests, and ending up with the long-term exhaustive carcinogenicity test which has as its pilot study various mutagenicity tests. This whole process will take more than five years of dedicated, intricate and painstaking work involving the handling and processing of thousands of blood samples to be tested for a variety of blood-cell and blood-chemistry parameters, and thousands of organ and other specimens, together with slides of animal tissues. All of these will be examined in detail and accurately reported upon. At the end of it, if nothing untoward is found there will be a reasonable prediction that the new medicine will be reasonably safe to use in man. Not a definitive prediction, only a reasonable one.

As we shall see later, this process of investigation will be augmented with human tests of increasing complexity and ever-lengthening timescales. In the middle and later stages both animal and human testing necessarily run in parallel because of the timescale involved.

5

Formulation Development

What is a *formulation*? Basically it is a carefully chosen combination of the active drug substance together with various other pharmacologically inert substances (but with useful physical properties). These latter substances enable the active ingredient to be delivered to the recipient and ensure it is available to the body for the intended use. Therefore the early establishment and development of an effective formulation is critical to the product's progress since the later clinical work will depend upon it. The formulation may also have an influence on the eventual success of the new medicine when it is marketed, since if it is unattractive for any reason the patient may not take it.

Although it has not been specifically mentioned so far, the marketing function of a pharmaceutical company does have an important input in to drug development at virtually all stages. Ideally it should be involved from the early days of compound selection, building up over the years so that when all the investigations have been done and the regulatory authorities have been satisfied (see later) marketing personnel will be really familiar with the actions of the new drug. This is important since the marketing function is one of the main links between a pharmaceutical company and the medical profession.

DIFFERENT TYPES OF PRESENTATION

There are literally dozens of different ways in which a new medicine can be formulated for use by the patient. In some instances the physical form of the new drug dictates to a large degree the formulation which is chosen. In the vast majority, however, the actual presentation will be derived to satisfy both technical and marketing considerations.

The most obvious difference in form is between liquid and solid. Sometimes a substance may only exist as a liquid. If this is so it could be administered by mouth either alone or with suitable diluting agents, or in liquid-filled capsules. Alternatively it could be administered as drops for the eye or ear. It may be intended to administer it by injection. Injections are commonly given intravenously or intramuscularly (rarely intrathecally, i.e. into the space surrounding the spinal cord). Whichever route of injection is intended, the substance should

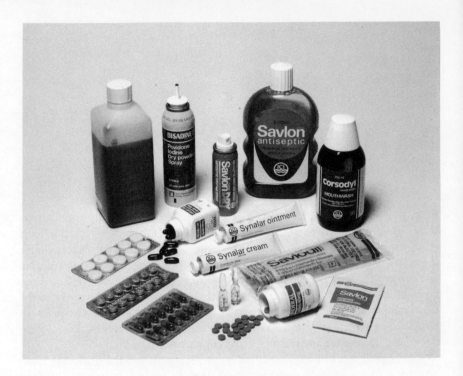

Figure 29 A group of some of the many different formulations, including solutions, tablets, capsules, creams and ointments, and a dry-powder spray.

be non-irritant. It is clearly undesirable either to irritate a vein so that it becomes painful and may become blocked, or to produce an abscess with an irritant intramuscular injection. Furthermore, such adverse reactions are extremely unlikely to help the bioavailability of the drug. For the drug to be presented as an injection it must have acceptable absorption characteristics and these will have been worked out during the pharmacodynamic and pharmacokinetic experiments on animals already described above. The presence or absence of irritancy will also have been investigated and identified during toxicology studies in animals, and the results will have been made available to the formulation scientists so that any required modifications can be carried out. Of course the release characteristics of such injectable formulations (as with *all* formulations) will need to be confirmed in man using both single and multiple doses (*see* chapter 6, Human Pharmacology).

In practice, however, most new drug substances exist as solids which can either be dissolved in various liquids to produce an injectable form or used as a solid dosage form (or both if the situation requires it). Solid dosage forms are commonly encountered as capsules, tablets, suppositories and pessaries.

Sometimes it may be impossible to produce a solution for injection. While this will preclude usage as an intravenous injection, an intramuscular injection as a suspension may still be possible. Of course, a suspension may also be given by mouth. For substances with unusual solubilities it may be necessary to administer them as an emulsion or in soft gelatine capsules which will contain a non-aqueous solution.

Undoubtedly therefore most new medicines are presented as tablets or capsules. Such capsules are usually of the hard gelatine kind (as opposed to the soft gelatine capsules already mentioned above), which have a number of advantages. They can be used where it is desired to mask the taste of a compound and

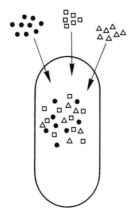

Figure 30 A capsule can be filled with a number of different types of granule, which may contain different medications with different 'time-release' characteristics.

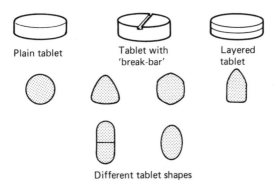

Figure 31 Developments from the plain round tablet are shown. They include tablets with break-bars to permit divided dosage and different tablet shapes to establish product identity. Different medicines can be co-administered in the same tablet, using a layered presentation.

also have an advantage where the physical form of the compound is such that it does not permit effective compression into a tablet. The substance can still be given orally without resorting to the perhaps slightly less convenient oral suspension. Capsules have further advantages in terms of size compared with dosage volume since as a rule they contain only very limited quantities of excipients (the non-pharmacologically active components of the pharmaceutical formulation). They also enable a mixture of drugs to be given at one time which may have different release characteristics. To achieve this the capsule is filled with two or three different types of granules in a set proportion which produce the desired pharmacological actions. If this were not possible it would necessitate taking two or three different types of tablets. Capsules also provide a readily apparent product identification (black and green, red and black, etc) and can aid the marketing function in providing a medicine which is attractively coloured and presented. Naturally they have a few disadvantages. The most important is that of expense since apart from the cost of the hard gelatine capsule shell itself the rate of capsule filling is much slower than can be achieved with tablet production. They also suffer from the drawbacks of impossibility of division of dosage (no one can take half a capsule) and where some people are concerned may present difficulties in swallowing.

Tablets, on the other hand, which can be produced in a bewildering variety of shapes and colours, being much quicker to produce are far cheaper. They offer the possibility of divided dosage when provided with break bars, and also if manufactured as layered tablets can permit the co-administration of fast and slow release forms of either the same agent or different agents. Indeed they can enable even chemically incompatible substances to be co-administered in the same tablet.

They have a slight disadvantage when product identity is concerned because of current regulations concerning the addition of colouring matter to medicines. Only a few dyes are currently permissible (and the list is diminishing) and so product identity by this means is more limited than with capsules. However, this can be relatively easily overcome by the adoption of different characteristic tablet shapes (e.g. triangular, pentagonal, heptagonal, etc).

FORMULATION COMPONENTS

A formulation normally consists of the active agent mixed with a number of pharmacologically inactive substances. These pharmacologically inactive substances are added to the formulation for a number of reasons such as to facilitate tableting or to maintain release characteristics of the medicine. Accordingly excipients can be included which may be binding agents or disintegrating agents (see below) while other substances will be present as lubricants or fillers. The latter type of substance will be extremely important if the new medicine is very potent since if the daily dose is discovered to be only 0.5 mg, a tablet of this weight, or even a very few multiples of it, would be totally impracticable. A filler

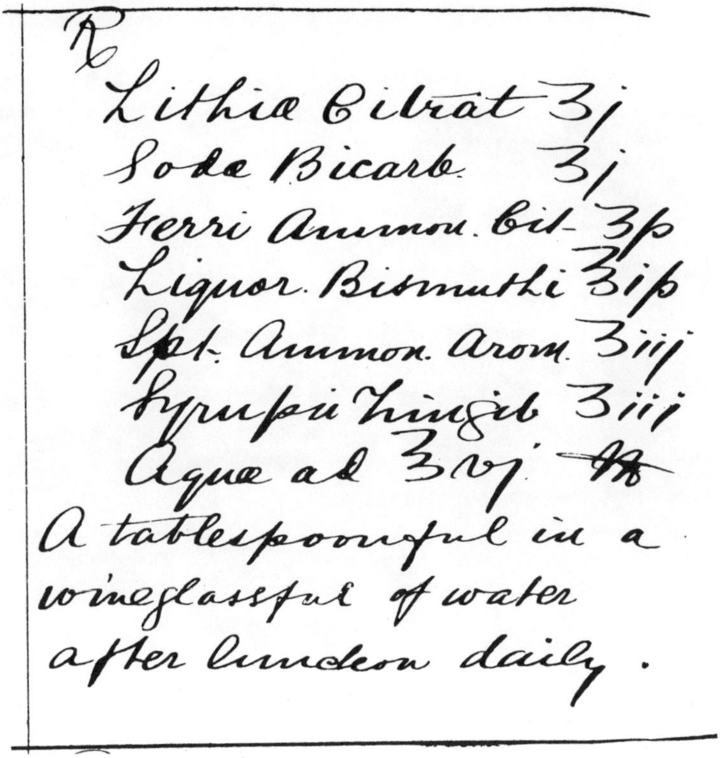

> ℞
> Lithia Citrat 3j
> Soda Bicarb. 3j
> Ferri Ammon. Cit. 3p
> Liquor. Bismuthi 3ip
> Spt. Ammon. Arom. 3iij
> Syrupu Zingib 3iij
> Aqua ad 3vj.
> A tablespoonful in a
> wineglassful of water
> after luncheon daily.

Figure 32 A modern formulation is often a complex affair but scientifically logical. This contrasts starkly with old formulations such as this nineteenth century example.

is therefore added. The mixing process then becomes important since it will be necessary to ensure that 0.5 mg of the drug is evenly dispersed in each and every tablet.

TABLET COATING

Tablets can be produced either in the uncoated form or they may have a film or sugar coat. Sugar coating, which was very much in vogue some years ago, has now been very largely superseded by film coating. Originally sugar coating was designed to mask the taste of a compound. It is rapidly becoming obsolete because it is a many-stage process and therefore expensive. It is also difficult to control from batch to batch. The process is somewhat messy and other cleaner, neater and more controllable methods have taken its place.

Film coating has a number of obvious advantages. First of all it can confer a significant degree of protection to the product, protecting it from the effects of moisture, oxidation and light. This is particularly important if the new medicine is light and moisture sensitive since if it cannot be guaranteed to be

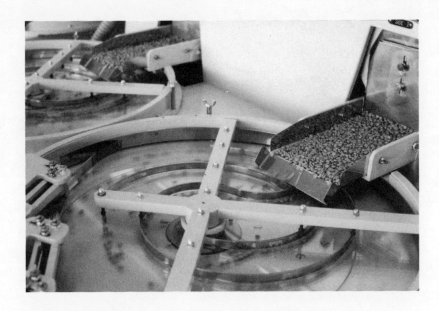

Figure 33   Recently produced tablets are mechanically 'organised' prior to packaging.

stable for a suitable period of time (see below) its future utility may well be
jeopardised. To aid this protective function various opacifying agents can be
added to the film-coating material. Film coating will provide additional tablet
strength thereby preventing chipping when tablets are moved around the factory
in bulk or indeed packaged in bulk for later dispensing by pharmacists. As with
sugar coating, it can be used to mask a bitter or unpleasant taste (or indeed the
effects of the medicine if it has a local anaesthetic effect in the mouth) and it
will aid swallowing. Furthermore, a film coat could perhaps be used to alter
drug release characteristics, and finally it can be used as a vehicle to add colour
to the tablet.

Film coating is judged to be better than sugar coating because it permits an
increased throughput of tablets, decreases product variability, and decreases
labour costs and factory space requirements. Having said this, however, there
are some concomitant disadvantages. It is expensive in terms of a high capital
cost and there are problems of solvent recovery and the flame-proofing of the
production area to safeguard against the spread of fire. In addition it is extremely
difficult to re-work poorly produced tablets. This will result in an increased

material cost which may be important if the drug is very expensive to produce. Furthermore, the process requires a significant amount of skill to carry it out and there are many things that can go wrong. Tablets can be subject to blistering, chipping, cracking, wrinkling and flaking, and many other defects. All of this will not only spoil the look of the product, but could influence the release characteristics.

TABLET CORES

Having made these observations about film coating and sugar coating, it is perhaps worthwhile to look briefly at how the tablet cores which will be so treated are manufactured in the first place. Basically there are three methods of producing tablet cores. The first is slugging which is rapidly becoming obsolete and therefore will not be considered further. This leaves two major methods and obviously the easiest is that of straightforward direct compression of the formulation into a tablet. If this is not possible because of the physical characteristics of the material, the new chemical entity can be converted to granules using either a wet or dry technique. Having produced the granules it is then possible to compress these into a tablet. As an extension of this, layered tablets incorporating one or two layers can be produced which might either have the function of incorporating fast or slow release forms of the same chemicals, or indeed might permit two incompatible (from the tableting point of view) active ingredients to be given at the same time.

To summarise the above, if the new chemical is susceptible to formulation as tablets the dosage strengths are selected early on in the development process. In fact it is often a guess, because it will be before clinical testing has started, and is based on animal work. If the dose is a small one and the material is stable then it is possible that the tablet core may be produced by direct compression of the material. On the other hand, if dosage size is in the medium range, direct compression may still be possible but granulation may need to be considered. With regard to high dosage compounds, granulation methods (either wet or dry) are usually chosen. Irrespective of how the cores are produced, they will be subject to testing for moisture sensitivity (here a wet granulation would be inappropriate), compressibility and friability.

Nowadays the technology involved in producing and controlling the quality of tablet cores is extremely complex. An extensive amount has been learnt over many years about the tensile strength of such cores as various materials have been empirically tabletted. Tablets can of course be too hard, too soft and subject to breaking up at the edges and corners, or indeed to cracking around their circumference (capping). All of these defects are clearly unacceptable. They present problems which may take many hours of detailed work to resolve. The characteristics of the tablet in terms of hardness, softness, etc may well have an important bearing on bioavailability of the active component.

SPECIAL PRESENTATIONS

So far we have mainly concentrated on (hard gelatine) capsules and tablets, and have mentioned injections. As described above, many additional presentations are possible. For paediatric use syrups and suspensions may be preferred, suitably flavoured. Other medicines are dispensed as powders (analgesics) or as gels (antacids). Again there is the whole range of ointments and creams for topical usage, and of course suppositories, pessaries and even implants may be required. Subject to specialised development are medicines intended to be administered directly to the lungs, which may be dispensed as powders and aerosols. Not only do these have their own particular problems of formulation and manufacture, but also the whole course of preclinical and clinical investigation is highly complex.

Whatever the final form or forms of the new medicine, the formulation will effectively consist of an active ingredient, coupled with various inactive agents which are incorporated either to maintain the integrity of the formulation in its preferred dosage form or to permit easier and more accurate working of the formulation during the course of manufacture of the finished product.

PRODUCT STABILITY

Therefore one of the most important aspects of any formulation is to ensure that it remains stable throughout the life of the product and that it is not subject to breaking down into either less active or more toxic decomposition products. The pure substance and the final form (tablets, capsules, etc) are therefore tested for their stability characteristics. The pure substance alone is usually tested at 37°C and 50°C and also at 37°C under high humidity conditions (75% relative humidity). The finished product will be subject to such testing at 4°C, 25°C, 25°C (high humidity), 37°C and 37°C (high humidity). The latter series (finished product) is tested for its storage characteristics in different packs and containers (such as glass bottles, polystyrene bottles, blister packages, etc) because the finished product may be stable in one form of pack (such as glass bottles) but interact unfavourably with polystyrene, for example. If, on the other hand, it is stable in all three forms, it gives marketing departments more freedom with regard to the eventual presentation to be marketed. The object of this stability testing is to provide guidance with regard to shelf life not only in temperate climates but also in those countries subject to more extreme conditions. It will give a guide to what might happen if the bottle is opened and closed many times in, say, a humid climate. Both the pure substance and the finished product are assayed for degradation products using various sophisticated methods. In addition, whether or not the product needs to be protected from light will have been assessed. The tablets will also be tested at regular intervals not only for appearance, but also for maintenance of hardness and disintegration, dissolution and friability characteristics. Therefore when a company claims

a product remains stable for five years, its opinion is based on factual knowledge.

PACKAGING

Before leaving this section the subject of packaging of pharmaceuticals should
perhaps be considered in a little more detail. Most people will be aware of the
circumstances surrounding the interference with Tylenol recently in the USA
where the final pack was interfered with and cyanide introduced maliciously
into the capsules by a member of the public. This has drawn the attention to the
necessity for adequate security of the product once it leaves the pharmaceutical
manufacturer's premises and various forms of tamper-proof packaging have been
developed as a result. This has also had the unexpected(?) benefit of reducing
pilferage of the product. Another aspect of security though is that of child
safety and recently various forms of bottle-caps have been developed which
prevent easy access by children. However, they suffer from the drawback that
they are not always readily accessible to those who need the medicines (in
particular arthritis sufferers).

Unit packing (blisters) has become very much in vogue recently since although
it adds slightly to the expense, it does permit non-interference or obviates the
risk of cross-contamination with other tablets in the pack, and in the case of
oral contraceptives enables a ready account to be made of how many tablets have
actually been taken. Unit packing and various security containers confer a degree
of protection on the drug in terms of extending its shelf life. When attractively
produced it can also be a significant marketing aid and reinforce the product's
identity.

The question of formulation development has been dealt with here for the chief
reason that the earlier the final formulation is arrived at the better for the development of any new product. All of the subsequent work can be directly related
to this final formulation, and will therefore be directly relevant to the subsequent marketing of the product. Since all of the human work from phase I
onwards (see later) will seek to prove the efficacy of the new compound, it is
as well to be sure that it can actually be formulated in the physical form it is
desired to market it in, that that physical form is stable, that it can be manufactured in the quantities likely to be required and that degradation products do
not arise as a result of moisture, light or oxygen, or as a result of excipients
introduced into the formulation. Therefore the earlier all this can be settled the
better. But there is another reason, and that is that although there are various
forms of accelerated storage tests currently in use in pharmaceutical development, the longer these storage tests have actually been running the better in
terms of definitively proving that the new medicine has the shelf life that the
manufacturers would wish to claim for it.

It should not be imagined that this whole area of formulation development running through to mass production is a quick one. It is fraught with problems which arise intercurrently during the course of development, for example it may be perfectly feasible to produce tablets on a hand press singly or indeed on one of the slower presses, but it may be totally impossible to get the formulation to run at the required rate of, say, five thousand or six thousand tablets per minute. Solving these many and detailed problems will take possibly three or four years and perhaps even longer. It goes without saying that the earlier the process is started the better.

6
Human Pharmacology

The compound has now been identified and subjected to animal pharmaco-logical investigation followed by initial animal toxicology work. Considering all of the results so far it is established that the new medicine appears to have interesting activity, which in the opinion of the researchers should be followed up rapidly by investigation in man. The key to successful development is to try the compound in man as soon as possible in the course of its development. Although animal tests do have a predictive value they do not provide any abso-lute degree of predictability, and therefore the only way of being sure that the compound has suitable utility and safety in man (and that it is not differentially toxic to man, for instance) is to proceed to human pharmacology. Furthermore there is an additional benefit because the information gained from human pharmacology studies might be utilised to alter the design of the chemical so that it more efficiently fits the human need.

The sooner the human pharmacology experiments are performed, particularly as we shall see with regard to metabolism studies, the sooner it will be possible to select the most appropriate animal species for the long-term toxicity studies.

It is generally accepted that as a minimum before the medicine is given to humans a 14-day toxicity study in animals should have been carried out. This will be performed at three dosage levels and with a control group as already described. Assuming that there is sufficient separation between the low dose in this toxicity experiment and the high dose (which will produce some degree of animal toxicity), and that the supposed human effective dose falls somewhere between this range (which should approximate much more closely to the lowest dose than the upper end of the scale), a decision can be taken to proceed to man. Another way of looking at this is to say that whatever the limitations of the LD 50 and ED 50 there should ideally be a wide separation between the two. At this very early stage, dose selection may be somewhat empirical. The rule is to commence cautiously with small doses (about one tenth of the expected average human dose), which are then either increased or decreased depending on the observed effects.

HUMAN VOLUNTEERS

Patients, i.e. humans with the particular condition that the new medicine is designed to affect, are not involved at this stage. The new medicine is tested first in normal and fit volunteers who cannot be said to be deriving any clinical benefit from the new substance. They are in fact volunteering because of their interest in the development of new medicines. Volunteers or not, their interests still have to be protected and therefore before any human-volunteer pharmacology studies are performed the protocols for such studies should be considered by an Ethics Review Committee composed of both doctors and lay personnel, which will ensure that the necessary safeguards are present to prevent foreseeable permanent damage to individuals' health.

Individuals are selected on the basis of having been previously healthy and are examined both physically and biochemically to confirm that this is indeed the case. Before commencing their participation in the study the nature of the experiment is carefully explained to them and they may indeed be asked to sign a form testifying to the fact that the procedure has been explained and that they have understood the risks (informed consent – see later). Of course the risks at this stage are largely speculation since nothing is known about the compound's behaviour in humans and knowledge extrapolated from animals may have no bearing whatsoever on either short- or longer-term effects.

Human pharmacology is directed firstly towards establishing the pharmacokinetics of the new compound so as to provide information on its bioavailability for a range of different doses. Secondly it is directed to determining whether the pharmaco-dynamic profile of the new agent is similar to that which has been previously demonstrated in animals. Thirdly it is directed towards assessing both local (i.e. by injection and also gastric) and general degrees of tolerance. Therefore the studies are in part confirmatory of the animal findings and in part extend our knowledge of the compound.

CORRELATION OF ANIMAL AND HUMAN FINDINGS

If the result of the pharmacokinetics studies is a true positive it will confirm the animal pharmacological findings and will provide the company with a number of perhaps not very exciting but nonetheless definite leads arising from already established compounds. With this sort of finding it is difficult to break new ground. If the findings have been negative or marginal in animals and this is confirmed in man then this is a true negative result and it closes an avenue of pharmacological investigations of either one or a series of compounds. Sometimes, however, false positives arise in so far that an effect is identified in animals, but activity in man is nil. Here it may be that activity resides in a part of the molecule which is handled differently by animals and man. By characterisation of this difference it may be possible to identify an agent with unusual activity in both animals and man. Through this process human pharmacology may offer a chance to create a real lead or even a new avenue of research. A false negative where an interesting effect in animals is not confirmed in man for 'false' or obscure reasons is a bad result since it may lead to the loss of good compounds. The false negative is the most important of the variables from the pharmacologists' point of view and naturally every effort is taken to circumvent it.

The area of true and false positives and negatives is an interesting one. In some contrast to the pharmacologists' standpoint, a true positive result in toxicology is not popular because it closes down that particular compound's progress. However, it may be possible to redeem the situation by modifying the chemical development pathway before too much time and money have been expended. However, it may be psosible to redeem the situation by modifying the chemical molecule without affecting therapeutic activity. On the other hand, a true negative result although disheartening for the pharmacologist is an excellent result to the toxicologist. In today's milieu, however, it requires real confidence to believe it fully. A false positive in toxicological terms is a bad outcome because a useful compound may be abandoned for the wrong reasons. Worse still, however, is a false negative result which could expose humans to serious risk.

HUMAN PHARMACOKINETICS

Turning now to the human pharmacokinetic investigations, the major elements to be established are first of all how the compound is absorbed and then how rapidly this occurs. Other questions to be answered are how it is distributed around the body, how it is metabolised and how it is excreted? The metabolism and excretion questions are extremely important in terms of yielding significant additional information for the future orientation of the long-term animal work still to be done. Obviously the long-term animal (toxicology) studies will be much more meaningful if the routes of metabolism and excretion in the species selected are the same or similar to those found in man.

A group of, say, six male volunteers is assembled, all having been previously vetted for robust good health and absence of inappropriate intemperate habits. After careful clinical and biochemical examination they are organised into groups of, say, three and given single doses of the compound. The dose selected is the lowest dose which would be expected to produce some activity in man based upon the findings in animals described hitherto.

Studies done on human volunteers are done under carefully supervised conditions usually in a 'hospital-type' setting under close medical and nursing supervision and with all equipment available to prevent or ameliorate a catastrophe should this occur. By using two groups of three 'patients', the dosage can be increased by weekly intervals using alternate groups, and the analysis of the serial blood samples taken during the experiments can be available for consideration before proceeding further.

Before commencing the experiment the volunteers are prepared in a standard fashion so that the drug is taken on an empty stomach and during the course of the day's observation only standardised fluids (i.e. water) and meals are taken.

A blood sample as a baseline is obtained and subsequent samples are taken at frequent intervals following the administration of the dose in order to ascertain how quickly the material is absorbed, and by plotting the analysis of the samples, how quickly it rises to a peak concentration in the blood, and how quickly it is thereafter removed. During the course of these investigations the volunteers are carefully observed and any untoward clinical signs are recorded and investigated, as are the ECG and blood chemistry. The function of all systems (such as the central nervous system and the respiratory system) is monitored at intervals throughout the duration of the study.

As these experiments proceed it will become apparent that either there is no effect, in which case after consideration the dosage is increased, or indeed if there is an effect, and that effect having been quantified, the dosage may still be increased to ascertain whether increments of dosage produce enhanced effects which may be either good or bad. The aim of these experiments will be to identify whether there is a separation between the supposed effective (thera-peutic) dose and the observation of any toxicity. They will also establish whether a dose–effect relationship exists and if so what type it is.

By using serial blood samples and suitable analytical techniques, the absorp-tion, distribution, metabolism and excretion of single doses can be worked out. This information when fed into a computer model will allow prediction of the likely time interval to achievement of a steady state, i.e. where absorption balances out metabolism and excretion. The steady state is commonly con-sidered as being achieved after five half-lives, a half-life being that time at which half an administered dose is still available to the body. Half-lives can vary enor-mously from only a minute or two to three or four days and beyond. Of course, using different formulations the half-life of a new medicine can be either shortened or extended.

Having done these absorption/distribution/metabolism/excretion (ADME for short) studies of single dosage, the next step would be to proceed to multiple dosage repetition at which the length of time required to achieve the steady state would be absolutely worked out (guided by the computer prediction). Also of course, prior to this experiments would have been done to compare and contrast the distribution curves of the new compound in the human body after both oral and intravenous dosage. The latter has the obvious advantage that it is known (once the injection is complete) that all of the dose is actually in the blood stream. Complete distribution of this will be achieved in about 25 heartbeats after which it starts to be removed by the body either by simple excretion or metabolism, or both. Whereas the intravenous dosage curve will start high and decline over time, the oral curve starts from nil, climbs to a maximum and then declines. For any human dose the 'area under the curve', i.e. the total amount present in the body during the experiment, should be approximately the same.

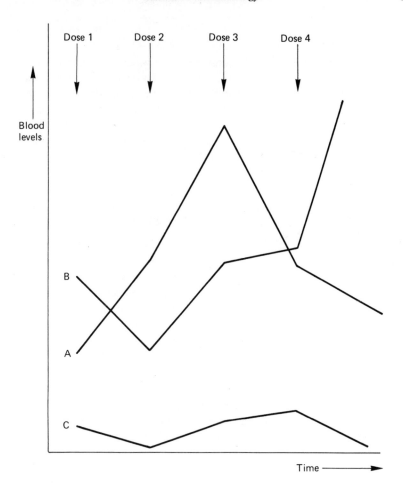

Figure 34 Showing what can happen in three ostensibly comparable and normal individuals given the same dose of a drug at the intervals shown. Subject A shows increasing levels until metabolism becomes established, when the levels begin to fall; subject B is clearly accumulating the drug; while subject C does not appear to be absorbing the drug effectively. (Redrawn from Conney *et al.*, *Clinical Pharmacology and Therapeutics*, University Park Press, 1980.)

If this is not the case then it is possible that the compound will not have been effectively absorbed via the alimentary tract. If and when this occurs the reasons for it must be investigated and established. Alternatively, if, for instance, there were differences in metabolic capability within the volunteer group, not only would the areas under the curves not be the same, but also the pharmacologically observed effects might be different. Of more practical importance in patients is the fact that a significant proportion of the population has a deficiency in oxidative metabolic processes. This can affect handling of a new drug in a variety of ways. For instance, many drugs are active in the parent form but inactive as metabolites. If metabolism is inefficient more active drug will be present in the patient's body after unit dosage. If we are depending on oxidative metabolism as with a 'pro-drug', the absence of metabolism might mean that there is no therapeutic effect or indeed metabolism may be a necessary step prior to efficient excretion. Thus there is either accumulation and overdosage on the one hand or lack of efficacy on the other. Furthermore, the absence of a 'normal' metabolic process may lead to unusual effects due to mediation through alternative enzyme systems. It is preferable if at least an early view of such factors can be obtained before involving patients, but in any event the studies will need to be repeated in patients to ensure completeness of the results or to identify possible differences.

Thus at the end of these carefully monitored studies the following information will have been generated:

- What likely human therapeutic dose is established as being reasonably safe to be given to patients? (Reasonably safe because it cannot be definitively so established until it has been given to patients.)
- A tolerated dose range will be known and the quantities which will produce different toxic effects in man will have been identified.
- The characteristics of absorption, whether through the stomach or lower down in the intestine, will be known and may point the way towards the need for a different formulation.
- The metabolism and excretion pattern will be known and indeed early information will be available on whether this is different for single or multiple dosing and different between individuals.
- With regard to toxicity or intolerance, the target organ or organs, e.g. heart, respiratory tract or central nervous system, will have been identified. Hopefully there will be a significant separation between that dose which would be expected to produce a therapeutic effect while not producing a toxic effect. However, in some compounds these limits of tolerance may be extremely narrow (e.g. digitalis) and it is important that this early knowledge of how to use the drug in practice is carefully sifted and evaluated, otherwise therapeutically important compounds might be abandoned unjustifiably.
- Possibly most importantly, the metabolic and excretory route (or routes) used by man will have been identified, which can be used to such telling effect in the design and carrying out of further animal toxicity work.

Thus human pharmacology is an essential step in determining first of all whether a compound should be progressed at all, and secondly if it is decided to progress a compound, to provide the critical information on which all future animal-safety (toxicology), human-safety and efficacy studies depend.

THERAPEUTIC PREDICTABILITY

It must also be recognised that with some classes of new drug, predictability of therapeutic effects from animal (and indeed human) pharmacology work is virtually impossible (e.g. drugs for Parkinson's disease or anti-schizophrenic agents). However, with others (such as antibiotics where the minimum inhibitory concentration of the drugs related to the bacteriological investigations can be plotted), predictability is good. Indeed, with some areas of medicine where, for instance, it is desired to test in human volunteers a new anti-asthmatic drug, the effects of the new drug on artificially induced bronchospasm of various types can be accurately evaluated. Therefore the scope and utility of the human pharmacology work will be governed by the area of medicine in which the compound is active. Even if this is not possible, the utility of the information on human tolerance and pharmacokinetic performance is self-evident.

ADDITIONAL STUDIES

Human volunters are also used at other stages in the drug development process for various confirmatory studies. One of these occurs when it is desired to check the supposed metabolic and excretion pathway of a new drug by a more sophisticated technique. This usually involves giving a dose of the new drug which has been made radioactive with C 14 or some other radio-isotope and carefully measuring its absorption, distribution, metabolism and excretion in the human body. For obvious reasons, such studies are usually done in males who (for all practical purposes) have passed through the reproductive phase of their lives and who are 'middle-aged'.

Another area in which human volunteers are employed is in bioavailability studies of various forms. These experiments are designed to confirm whether a new formulation of a tablet, capsule, suppository or other dosage form is comparable to formulations previously used in what might have been extensive clinical studies. If comparability is demonstrated then it may be reasonably concluded that the new formulation will perform equally as well as the old version. When the formulation is changed, and this may be for a variety of reasons, such a study must be performed because it cannot be presumed that a new formulation will perform equivalently or better than the old one.

SPECIAL STUDIES

Finally there is the use of human volunteers in various special types of study. For example, it is known that anti-arthritic preparations (non-steroidal anti-inflammatory — NSAI — agents) of various types and classes will produce a degree of blood loss from the intestinal tract. With a new anti-arthritic agent the aim would be to investigate whether this blood loss is comparable to other commonly prescribed agents or whether it is better or worse. Volunteers are given a small dose of radioactive chromium (Cr 51) which is attached (tagged) to a sample of their red blood cells which has been withdrawn from a vein. The fate of these cells when re-injected into the original donor is then plotted using their radioactivity as a marker. The study involves taking the drug or drugs under test, removing blood samples and collecting faecal material over a number of days (usually about fourteen). Although it is somewhat unpleasant it is nonetheless deemed a necessary study. Since the results are directly comparable between patients and volunteers it is the latter who are usually investigated to spare ill patients further nuisance.

Before going on to consider the great variety of true clinical studies it must be emphasised that human pharmacology (phase 1) work is virtually a hub around which successful development can and does turn. It can provide essential guidance to the chemists and pharmacologists for improvements and modifications of chemical molecular design. Information is supplied to the toxicologists for species selection for further studies and indeed these key data on drug handling are necessary for the formulators to be sure of their formulation. Looking forwards, it establishes the bedrock for proceeding cautiously towards obtaining the answer to the question 'what is the efficacy/safety profile in the patient?'.

7

Evaluation of Human Efficacy and Safety

Although the new drug can fail for various reasons during the stages in its progress so far described, the next phase, that of clinical evaluation, is undoubtedly the most critical. Until efficacy at a defined dose or doses is established in the actual patient population which the drug candidate has been designed for, together with an acceptable safety profile, the drug candidate cannot move along the pathway leading to its eventual registration as a significant product.

Like the chronic toxicity studies, clinical evaluation should be started as soon as possible since it will run for at least three to four years (and with some drugs for much, much longer) before registration. Of course, clinical work (either confirmatory of existing work or alternatively exploring new actions and indications) is virtually always in progress even long after registration for the original indication has been granted in a number of territories. It lasts for as long as the product is used by man.

The clinical phase will commence with the knowledge that, in short-term toxicity studies at any rate, the compound does not appear to be unduly harmful in animals. The early formulation studies will have indicated that it is capable of at least being dispensed in a simple formulation as previously described, although the marketing function may well want something more sophisticated for a variety of reasons, and indeed a more sophisticated presentation may be predicted as the clinical studies proceed. Human pharmacology will have indicated that in single and multiple doses the compound appears to be relatively safe in normal man. As described, depending upon the area of medicine the new drug is designed for, there may or may not be early evidence of efficacy in human volunteers. For instance, this may be more readily predicted with a broncho-dilating (relaxing) agent (when broncho-constriction can be artificially produced) than with a drug deemed to be useful in combating schizophrenia. Additionally such studies will have generated some dose-ranging information in relation to effects on other body systems besides the one that the drug is primarily designed to affect.

This critical phase of clinical development starts, as with all others, very simply and builds up in complexity as the development programme proceeds. There is a singular difference between this and the preceding phase of human pharmacology in that the new drug is now being used for the first time in humans actually suffering from the condition it is designed to treat, i.e. these people are ill in varying degrees. It is perhaps unfortunately the case that when a new medicine is promulgated it often tends to be tried in the initial phase at least by those people who have failed to benefit from all of the other medicines previously available. It has been argued that this is perhaps too stringent a test for a new medicine especially when the profession is in the very early stages of learning how to use it. However, for a variety of reasons this is usually how a potential new medicine starts its clinical life. Often, with severely afflicted patients (for example, whether in severe pain or with severe degrees of hypertension) the new drug is increased in dosage to produce an acceptable level of efficacy and while this is proceeding an excessive side-effect level may be demonstrated. It then becomes the task of the clinical researcher to design less stringent experimental conditions to define more closely the efficacy/unwanted effect ratio in a much wider variety of patients. The importance of this type of start up is the recognition that while a new drug may not be dramatically effective in this most seriously afflicted population, it is not necessarily a useless agent for a whole variety of less severely affected patients.

CLINICAL TRIAL DEFINITION

In a Pharmaceutical Industry Working Party Report issued in 1974 a clinical trial was defined as 'a scientific experiment in which a drug or procedure is applied with diagnostic, therapeutic or prophylactic intent to patients. It is part of clinical pharmacology but stresses the clinical benefit.' This definition of a trial and the clinical-phase content of a whole series of clinical trials is still true today. What it is essentially saying is that a new medicine must not be given to a patient unless there is some reasonable expectation of benefit to the individual arising therefrom. Of course, as a result of these experiments information on safety will also be derived and this is obviously important for the future utility of the compound.

Alternatively, or additionally, a clinical trial may be defined as a carefully and ethically designed experiment which has the aim of answering a precisely framed question having therapeutic relevance. It is perhaps easier to be precise with the original question than it is to ensure that an investigator observes correctly all the criteria established beforehand to enable him to answer it effectively, or indeed that the patients will co-operate in the prescribed manner. Therein lie two of the major difficulties in clinical research. The fact that these difficulties exist, however, is not a valid reason for failing to ensure that the correct questions are posed.

CLINICAL PROGRAMME OBJECTIVES

The objective of this clinical trial phase or programme is therefore to produce direct answers to the following major questions:

- Indications for use. These must be defined so that the medical profession has a clear idea of when to use the new medicine and whom to use it on, i.e. which patient population with what condition will derive the most benefit.
- The programme will define the dosage range in the different indications. It will establish what the initial dose is and what the maintenance dose is for both the averagely affected and the severely affected patient.
- The actual method of usage of the dosage in ascending increments must be researched. Can the drug be introduced quickly or more slowly? Does this have different effects?
- It will establish the side actions or effects of the new medicine which may be beneficial as well as harmful and it will seek to quantify them and qualitatively define their degree.
- Of course patients in the less-well-controlled general-practice setting take a variety of medicines simultaneously. Therefore the possibility of drug interaction must be investigated. Some drugs will display antagonism, others will have additive effects while other different agents may exhibit true synergism. The majority of drugs will compete for plasma-protein binding sites and their effect or otherwise in this respect can and usually does affect the behaviour of other medicines the patient is taking.
- There is the question of different population groups. As a result of pharmaceutical research it has been established, for instance, that hypertension in the negro races is in many respects a different entity with regard to its response to treatment using currently available agents than hypertension in the white races. Again, orientals often display different metabolic propensities from occidental races. Therefore with respect to the international development of a new medicine, factors such as these must be identified and quantified if its activity and behaviour are to be fully understood (*see* Human Pharmacology earlier).
- Possibly as an extension of the comments above, there is the question of how the very young and very old will react to the new medicine. It is now a well-recognised fact that the young, for instance, cannot be regarded as small adults. Their behaviour and systems of handling a drug are often significantly different. Similarly, with the older patient, body systems are 'slowing down' and often they do not effectively metabolise a new agent. It can therefore accumulate and consequently produce toxic effects which are not seen in a younger population (see below).

PHASES OF CLINICAL RESEARCH

Certain areas of pharmaceutical drug development are beset by inexact terminology. The phase of human pharmacology already described is commonly referred to as phase I. All clinical studies are therefore designated as either phase II (early clinical research in which patient numbers are small and the degree of patient monitoring is very stringent) or leading on to phase III (following on as a logical extension of phase II to where patient numbers are being significantly expanded and monitoring by virtue of this is correspondingly much less), or phase IV which is that area of clinical research usually performed after the drug is registered and is being actively marketed and promoted. Many important facts can still be derived in phase IV (see later) and indeed it should be emphasised that as long as the drug is used by man, knowledge is never complete. New indications, new ways of using the new medicine and new populations who might benefit are continually being identified. Therefore this continuum of clinical research from phase II through phase III to phase IV will expand man's experience with the agent from only a few patients to perhaps thousands. While it is progressing there is also the question of additional pharmacokinetic work since it will be readily appreciated that patients with varying degrees of illness may handle the drug differently from those who are eminently healthy (volunteers), and who have provided the 'test-bed' for metabolism studies before clinical work was commenced.

RISK–BENEFIT PROFILE

The objective therefore in clinical research is essentially to establish the human dosage together with safety and efficacy at that dosage in the major conditions it is desired to treat. By this process the risk–benefit ratio should be carefully derived. There is no such thing as absolute safety. All drugs or procedures carry a risk. The risk may be small and definable but is a risk nonetheless. One of the prime objectives of a clinical programme is to try to define the risks. The degrees of risk which are acceptable in different situations will of course vary. If a condition is life threatening with the patient likely to die in any case, then even if the risk of using the medicine is high, it could nonetheless be an acceptable trade-off. If, however, the condition is relatively trivial, safety must be virtually absolute.

Interestingly, as an offshoot of this mainstream clinical programme there is often the identification of novel indications which are perhaps totally unrelated to the condition the new medicine has been designed for. Where this is the case the programme is started again from the human pharmacology phase and sometimes even further back, since it has to be intricately researched in the context in which it presents. Everybody, and especially the clinical researchers, should be constantly aware of the possibility of an unexpected finding since it may be that the drug's real utility lies with this rather than the initially designed and researched indication.

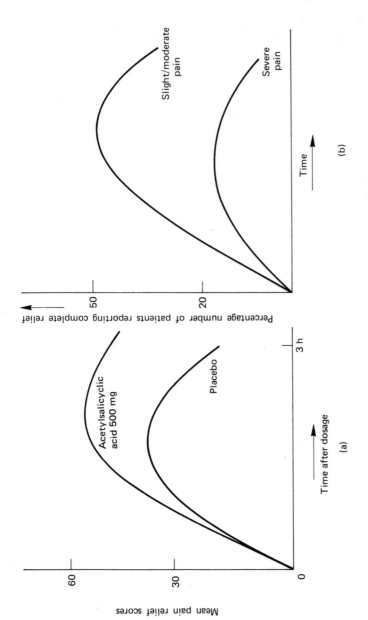

Figure 35 Placebos are powerful. In (a), although there is a significant difference between the active (acetylsalicylic acid) and placebo groups, nevertheless the placebo did provide a degree of analgesia. (b) shows that this was more likely to be the case in those with lesser degrees of pain (Redrawn from Lasagna, L., in *Therapeutic and Unwanted Effects: Drug Related or Not?*, 1978.)

TYPES OF CLINICAL TRIALS

Controlled or Uncontrolled

To accomplish this objective of definition of the risk–benefit ratio, distinct clinical trial designs are used which are appropriate in a variety of different medical conditions. One of the most important differences is whether the trial is controlled or uncontrolled. What this means is 'does the trial design incorporate some sort of known and reproducible baseline such as the concomitant study of a recognised comparator?'

Firstly, this comparator agent might be one of a number of other agents already established as of proven efficacy in the condition the new medicine is designed to affect.

Secondly, it could, however, be other forms of medical treatment but also, particularly in the early phases, it may consist of a *placebo*. This is a pharmacologically inert substance which therefore can have no effect pharmacologically although psychologically (because the recipient expects it to) it will have a demonstrable effect. Over the years there have been publications testifying to the potency of placebos in a number of situations which clearly indicate that they can, for instance, relieve pain at least over the short term and indeed can produce a variety of adverse and other reactions.

Thirdly, the comparison may be effected against a regime employing no treatment at all. Obviously, for effective and reproducible comparison all other variables in the experiment must be reduced as far as possible, e.g. time over which the study runs, nursing care and other conditions directly affecting the patients. It can readily be appreciated that a study examining the effects of a new anxiolytic could well be prejudiced in the event of a hospital strike. The object of 'control' by whatever means is to increase objectivity and reduce bias whether conscious or unconscious on the part of either the patient or the investigator.

The objective of all clinical research could be said to be based on disproving the 'null hypothesis'. In effect the research assumes at the outset that there is no difference between the two therapies and sets out to show that, in reality, there is a difference. The importance of ensuring that there are sufficient patient numbers to answer a clearly defined question without varying degrees of observer bias creeping in can therefore be clearly appreciated.

Open or Blind

Another important difference in trial design is whether it is completely open, which means that the physician knows exactly what he is giving and when, and that the patient knows he is either receiving a new medicine (which at any rate is expected to benefit his condition) or else a comparator, as above. These trials are usually employed in the early stages of investigation. However, they suffer from the important drawback of bias (conscious or unconscious) on the part of both physician and patient. To contrast this there can be various degrees of 'blindness' introduced into the clinical trial design. The simplest form is a single-blind study where the doctor will know that he is giving a new medicine but the patient will not know whether it is the new medicine, or an active comparator substance, or indeed a placebo, that he is receiving at any point in the course of

Medication Z = ○
Medication Y = ○

	Treatment period				
	1		**2**		
Patient 1.	Active Z Ⓐ	Placebo Y Ⓟ	Placebo Z Ⓟ	Active Y Ⓐ	
2.	Placebo Z Ⓟ	Active Y Ⓐ	Active Z Ⓐ	Placebo Y Ⓟ	
3.	Active Z Ⓐ	Placebo Y Ⓟ	Placebo Z Ⓟ	Active Y Ⓐ	
4. etc.	Placebo Z Ⓟ	Active Y Ⓐ	Active Z Ⓐ	Placebo Y Ⓟ	

(a)

Medication Z ○
Medication Y ○
Placebo △

	Treatment period		
	1	**2**	**3**
Patient			
1.	Active Z Ⓐ Dummy Y Ⓟ Placebo △	Dummy Z Ⓟ Active Y Ⓐ Placebo △	Dummy Z Ⓟ Dummy Y Ⓟ Placebo △
2.	Dummy Z Ⓟ Active Y Ⓐ Placebo △	Dummy Z Ⓟ Dummy Y Ⓟ Placebo △	Active Z Ⓐ Dummy Y Ⓟ Placebo △
3.	Dummy Z Ⓟ Dummy Y Ⓟ Placebo △	Active Z Ⓐ Dummy Y Ⓟ Placebo △	Dummy Z Ⓟ Active Y Ⓐ Placebo △

(b)

Figure 36 (a) Diagrammatic representation of testing two dissimilar medications in four patients double blind. To do this it is necessary to prepare identical placebos (dummies) for each active medication which are administered in a randomised way so that each patient only gets one active medication at a time. (b) A more complicated design, where it is considered necessary to incorporate a placebo to establish a baseline and where, for various reasons, it is impossible to match directly the two active medications.

the trial. Of course, where some medicines have distinct pharmacological/physiological actions and the comparator does not, it may be difficult to maintain blindness of the trial (e.g. testing a beta-blocking agent which will affect heart rate against a non-beta-blocking agent which does not). On the other hand, where a new drug has distinct actions on, say, the electrical activity of the heart (antidysrhythmics) a blind trial may not be strictly necessary as the ECG trace is an objective piece of evidence which hopefully cannot be 'fudged' by either patient or attending physician. This trial design can theoretically be worked the other way around, i.e. where the patient knew and the doctor did not, but in practice this would not be carried out unless, for instance, one was auditing a doctor's performance of trial activity. More complicated is a double-blind design where neither the patient nor the doctor knows who is getting what. This is done using two medications made to look identical and placed in identical cartons which are numbered in accordance with a list where the drugs are given in a completely randomised order. It enables, if the trial is properly carried out, a reasonable comparison to be made of the properties of the new agent with either an active comparator drug or a placebo. The attending physician is provided with a sealed code for the trial so that in the event of an emergency the code can be broken and the actual medication at any point in the trial for each and every patient can be determined. In practice it is important to get someone not closely associated with the trial to break the code; otherwise the integrity of the blinding of the trial with respect to the other patients could be jeopardised. Alternatively, individual codes for each patient can be prepared to obviate this risk.

Where two dissimilar medicines cannot be successfully matched for appearance, etc the pharmaceutical physician may resort to a 'double dummy' technique. This involves each agent having its own identical placebo comparator. It is more complicated since at each dosage interval the patient has to take two 'medications' instead of one (i.e. active test drug and inactive placebo comparator, or active comparator and placebo test drug). If this is impossible for any reason an 'observer blind' technique can be used where the medications are dispensed by a third party who takes no hand in the clinical assessment of the patients. The object of all these and other similar procedures is to eliminate, or at least greatly reduce, bias on the part of the attending physician and the patient. By removing bias there is more chance of getting at the truth.

PATIENT POPULATIONS

There are different patient populations to be used in these various clinical trial designs. The simplest is to establish a patient population which is treated with a new medicine and then proceeds to a comparator drug. This is a straight (within group) comparison design. It can be further refined in that the original patient population is divided into two groups, one of which gets the new medicine first (the other half the comparator) for a selected period of time, and the agent is then crossed over. By this design it is hoped to minimise any modification effect

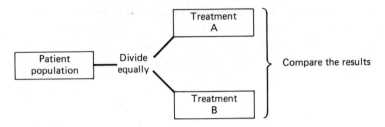

2 Groups—parallel design

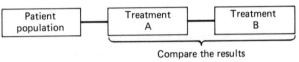

1 Group—sequential design

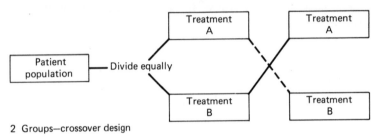

2 Groups—crossover design

Figure 37 Three methods of handling a patient population in comparative clinical trial design.

of the disease process which one or other of the agents might produce. This does have drawbacks, however, in assessing efficacy in either self-limiting conditions or when one or other agent is curative, or indeed alters the progress of the disease process. An example would be where a non-steroidal anti-inflammatory agent is compared with a gold or penicillamine-type of agent. These latter alter or modify the rheumatoid process so that the comparison could be invalidated.

An alternative way of comparing two treatments is to establish a patient population of matched pairs where patients are carefully matched in terms of age, gender, weight, disease severity, history and duration, etc and the two treatments are compared. However, this is a very lengthy procedure since it takes a long time to establish fairly accurately matched pairs of patients. Another method is to employ group comparisons where different groups of patients (as closely matched as possible) are used. Finally of course there are mixed designs where, for instance, matched pairs can be crossed over or even groups can be crossed over, etc.

This question of patient populations is an important one and during the phase of clinical investigation certain individuals are specifically excluded. Most importantly as a result of Thalidomide and other events, women of child-bearing potential, i.e. women who might get pregnant, may be eliminated from the trial population. Also those with certain allergic conditions and indeed those (in the early phases at any rate) with abnormal laboratory findings are specifically excluded. For each and every clinical trial there are certain categories of patients who are excluded mainly for two reasons. Firstly to remove the possibility of exposing patients who might be harmed, and secondly to exclude patients whose inclusion might cloud the validity of the study. As with the human pharmacology studies, the question of informed consent arises. It is essential that the patient knows exactly what is going to happen and what he or she might expect from participating in the study (see later). As a further safeguard for the patients, trials nowadays are subject to Ethics Committee review. These committees are composed of both professional and lay members and their agreement to the experiment is sought before carrying it out. In order that this can be done, the objective and nature of the experiment, together with a detailed plan of how it will be performed, must be available. This is stated in a protocol, and all clinical trials must be done to one.

THE PROTOCOL

This defines accurately what the intended experiment is, how it will be conducted and what the anticipated or likely outcome is expected to be. Protocol design considering all the different medical conditions it may be desired to treat or affect is an art in itself. Protocols are usually prepared by the pharmaceutical physician in charge of this part of the project and, on the basis that 'many heads are better than one', is subjected to detailed peer review by both physicians and other professional staff such as pharmacologists and statisticians. The latter have an important input 'before the fact' since the whole design of the experiment can have an important impact on the utility of the results in terms of their statistical validity. However, probably the most important aspect of the protocol is the definition of the question it is desired to answer, which experience dictates should be as simple as possible in order to afford the best chance of a clear result.

Ten years ago many trial protocols may have been only one or two pages long. They now extend to 20 or 30 pages and beyond, as areas of the trial which were previously based on an 'understanding' between clinicians and pharmaceutical physicians are closely and clearly defined. The clinical trial protocol will now specify the aim of the trial and the rationale for it. The experimental design (either a pure form or a combination of those mentioned above – which will be determined by the sensitivity of the experiment) will be declared and the numbers of patients required will be given. Those patients to be selected and those to be excluded will be defined, and the dosage, frequency and duration of therapy which those patients entering the trial will be expected to undergo are written out in full. The way in which the patients will enter the trial (randomisation or otherwise) and the various clinical and laboratory assessments (both the methods and their frequency) to be used to measure both the benefits and unwanted effects of the therapy, will be established. Frequently techniques are incorporated to check whether the patients are actually taking the mediciations as prescribed (i.e. patient compliance). This can be done by counting tablets remaining in the dispensary packs, blood sampling at given intervals or the incorporation of a marker (detectable in urine) within the clinical trial tablets. Finally the methods and degree of documentation for both physicians and patients are declared as is the mode of analysis of the results and the timescale for their presentation.

STATISTICAL INPUT

During the last decade particularly, statisticians have become increasingly involved in the prediction of the patient numbers which would be required to answer specific questions posed in the protocol. In the past, many trials have failed to answer the question asked (unfortunately for the wrong reasons) because either the patient numbers incorporated were inadequate to anwer the question within the limits of any statistical significance, or the wrong patients were selected. Another important area of involvement by statisticians and others, in particular computer personnel, is in the design of the patient record forms which may be for use either by the medical or ancillary staff, or by the patients themselves. Obviously the design of the form and the way in which the questions are set out will have a critical bearing on how accurately or otherwise the form is filled in. This in turn may well be critical to the success or failure of the study.

Clinical research has advanced greatly over the course of the last few years from being a relatively inexact science to one where increasingly stringent levels of professionalism are being incorporated. Even so, trials fail to produce the desired result in far too many instances. Some of the major reasons for failure are set out in table 7.1. The skill of the pharmaceutical physician is in many respects one of 'Jack of all trades', but in reality his specialist skills are paramount in this phase of development. They are just as important as those of a skilled toxicologist or a skilled pharmaceutical formulator to the successful development of a new medicine.

An important principle has been constantly referred to. This is the system of starting each main area of drug development simply. Simple experiments requiring simple answers are continually built up until the answers to many often very complicated questions are obtained. In this area of clinical research, the patient's welfare is of over-riding concern. Consequently, commencing from the very early stages, although the questions to be answered and the study design are simple, patient monitoring and supervision are not. At the outset patients are very elaborately monitored with regard to all bodily systems, and as knowledge and confidence builds, this is relaxed somewhat. It must be emphasised, however, that all patients are closely medically supervised in all stages of clinical research. If a physician considers that a patient is not benefiting during a clinical trial, that patient is usually withdrawn from the study.

**A COMPARATIVE STUDY OF CEFOTETAN
IN THE TREATMENT OF BACTERIAL INFECTIONS**

LABORATORY DATA I

| 1 | 5 | 6 | 8 | 3 | 4 | / | 7 | 0 | 0 | 2 | Visit Number | 0 5 | Centre Number | | Patient's Trial No. | | | A |

Patient's Identification

	Pre-Treatment	During Treatment	At Conclusion of Treatment	Follow-up (≃10 days after conclusion)
Date	20 D M Y	26 D M Y	32 D M Y	38 D M Y

Haematology

Was the differential WCC measured in:– (please tick) % 44 ☐ 1 $\times10^9$/l ☐ 2

	Pre-Treatment	During Treatment	At Conclusion	Follow-up
Total RCC $\times10^{12}$/l	45	49	53	57
Total WCC $\times10^9$/l	61	65	69	73
Polymorphs	77	81	85	89
Lymphocytes	93	97	101	105
Monocytes	109	113	117	121
Eosinophils	125	129	133	137
Basophils	141	145	149	153
Other cells	157	161	165	169
Platelets $\times10^9$/l	73	76	79	82

Differential WCC (normal / abnormal) (please tick)   85 ☐N ☐A   86 ☐N ☐A   87 ☐N ☐A   88 ☐N ☐A

Prothrombin Time

Enter value in seconds OR express as % of control value

Patient (secs)	89	92	95	98
Control (secs)	101	104	107	110
Patient %	113	116	119	122

Coombs test (if done) (positive / negative) (please tick)   125 ☐P ☐N   126 ☐P ☐N   127 ☐P ☐N   128 ☐P ☐N

Haematocrit %	129	131	133	135
Hb g/dl	137	140	143	146

Liver Function Tests

Total bilirubin	149	155	161	167
SGPT (ALT)	173	179	185	191
SGOT (AST)	197	203	209	215
Alkaline phosphatase	221	227	233	239
Serum Albumin	245	251	257	263

Renal Function Tests

Blood urea	269	275	281	287
Creatinine	293	299	305	311

COMMENTS

Signature: _____

Date: _____

Figure 38 (above and opposite) Two examples of fairly complicated record forms prepared for computer handling.

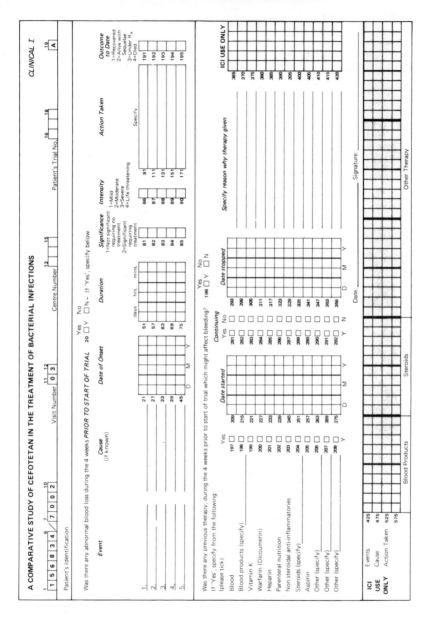

Table 7.1   Some causes of delay and failure to complete clinical studies

Faults in the . . .

Plan	e.g. protocol	Poor definition of questions Incorrect trial design Inadequate criteria for assessment
Powers	Ethics Committee Consultant Junior medical staff Nursing staff	Delay Loses interest Overworked Overworked, ineffectively briefed
Pilots	Pharmaceutical physician Clinical trials team Nurse observers	Inadequate monitoring Badly managed Badly motivated
Passenger	New drug	Inappropriate formulation Wrong dosage chosen Appearance of toxicity Inadequate clinical trials stock
Patients	Trial population	Badly selected Slow recruitment Inadequate numbers Unco-operative Not attending for assessments
Patient records	Data base	Badly designed forms Incompletely filled in Not properly identified Lost records
Pharmacists	Company Hospital	Faulty supply of material Faulty dispensing of materials
Publishing	New information	Incomplete results Poor writing-up Lack of impetus to publish

Adapted from Smith, R. B. (1976). Clinical trials – Phases II, III and IV, in *Principles and Practice of Clinical Trials* (Ed. C. S. Good), Churchill Livingstone

Note: The above list is by no means exhaustive. It does highlight, however, a degree of 'human frailty' which is often at the root of failure to plan, execute, analyse and publish the results of a clinical research experiment.

PHARMACOKINETICS IN PATIENTS

Apart from investigating, often during a number of years, efficacy and safety in an ever-expanding patient population, a number of other specific matters are considered during this clinical phase. Although human pharmacology will have given a good guide to the toxicologists regarding which particular animal species is best for their long-term experiments based on the closeness of that species' metabolism of the compound to man, the absorption, metabolism and distribution, and excretion of the compound may be different in patients as a whole or in various sub-groups of the patient population. Therefore some patients, after suitable information has been given and their informed consent has been obtained, will be involved in experiments to confirm this. They will also be involved in a whole variety of special studies in order to establish the handling of the drug in, for instance, patients with various degrees of liver or kidney failure. In addition, for example, effects on the skeletal system or calcium balance may be important. The list is almost endless and obviously will depend upon the exact nature of the new medicine being tested.

THE YOUNG AND THE ELDERLY

The initial clinical trial programme may specifically exclude two population groups – the young and the old – yet it may be that there are individuals in both groups who would benefit from the new treatment. Obviously both have to be specially investigated. It is a truism that children are not just small adults. They have a much larger surface area relative to body mass than adults, plasma protein binding capacity is lower, they have a higher extracellular fluid volume and, in the very young, drug metabolising enzymes may not have matured. All these and other differences ensure that special studies in children are necessary. However, they cannot give informed consent, and pharmacokinetic studies are extremely difficult.

Similarly, clinical research in the elderly is equally fraught with problems. Metabolism is slower and renal excretion is poorer. Absorption of drugs is probably less effective and more inconsistent than in younger adults, there is a reduced liver enzyme induction response and there may be increased volumes of distribution of drug within the body. All of this conspires to ensure that there are wide variations of response in an elderly population, but in general if standard adult dosing is employed, longer half-lives and higher plasma levels are observed. Furthermore, variability of response increases with age.

Both of these population groups will therefore be the subject of particular investigation either at a late stage of the pre-registration programme or indeed shortly after the first registrations have been granted.

INFORMED CONSENT

The giving of informed consent by both volunteers and patients alike has been mentioned a number of times. What this actually means is that the precise nature of the proposed experiment, the question it is designed to answer, the possible outcomes and the individual's part in the study are all carefully explained to the volunteer or patient by the physician sometimes in the presence of an impartial witness. Therefore the risks and possible benefits are enunciated and any questions that arise are answered. If the individual, now knowing more about what is intended, wishes to withdraw, this is possible without any degree of rancour or prejudice. If patients are involved, they should in no way be made to feel that the future conduct of their case will be prejudiced by their refusal to participate. On the other hand, if the patient or volunteer indicates his agreement to participate he must confirm that he has fully understood what is to occur and what is the likely outcome. He may be asked to sign a form confirming that a full explanation was given, he has completely understood it and is willing to participate of his own free will. Of course, it almost goes without saying that the true risks which obviously will not be known in a research situation cannot be foreseen and therefore explained. However, this fact does not preclude the necessity and duty to provide the patient or volunteer with the fullest and most balanced view possible of the possible outcomes before the experiment commences. The difficulty, though, of obtaining informed consent from certain population groups such as the young, very old or those with some mental conditions, can be readily appreciated.

CONFIDENTIALITY

Many patients invited to participate in phase II and phase III (or even phase IV) clinical trials may be concerned about confidentiality. Where all responsible pharmaceutical companies are involved they should not be unduly worried because security of information is a familiar discipline. In all clinical studies patients are codified by a number which can correspond to their hospital number. In consequence any clinical data included on the company's clinical trial record form is not directly identifiable back to that particular patient. If, for any reason, a patient needs to be identified by name, this is usually done in the first instance by contact between the company medical adviser and the patient's attending physician, whether from general or hospital practice. The majority of pharmaceutical companies are well versed in the necessity for security of information and confidentiality. Therefore this should not prove to be an area of concern for patients included in studies.

At the end of this clinical phase, however, all of the major aspects of drug development should come together so that the company will have a dossier

A COMPARATIVE STUDY OF CEFOTETAN
IN THE TREATMENT OF BACTERIAL INFECTIONS   *PATIENT INFORMED CONSENT*

| 1 | 5 | 6 | 8 | 3 | 4 | / | 7 | 0 | 0 | 2 | Visit Number | 0 | 1 | Centre Number | | | | Patient's Trial No. | | | | A |

Archive number   **156834/7002**   Centre number _____

                                                    Patient's trial number _____

Name of patient _____

Name of clinician _____

Consent obtained was:
(tick one box only)   (tick one box only)
                    20   21
          Written [ ] 1   Patient   [ ] 1
          Verbal   [ ] 2   Parent/Legal guardian [ ] 2

The nature of this study with cefotetan in the treatment of bacterial infections has been fully explained to me by
the above clinician. I hereby consent to take part in this study and I understand that I may withdraw from participation
in the investigation at any time.

                              Signature of patient _____

                                          Date _____

                              Signature of witness _____
                (when verbal consent ONLY is obtained)

                                          Date _____

                    Signature of parent/legal guardian _____
                          (when the patient is a minor)

                                          Date _____

I confirm that I have explained the nature of this study to the above named patient.

                              Signature of clinician _____

                                          Date _____

Figure 39 An informed consent form.

which, being compiled and presented to a number of government agencies, will permit registration of the new drug so that it can be effectively prescribed by the medical profession. As we have seen, however, clinical interest on the part of the company does not fade out at this point, but rather it intensifies (see later).

8

The Regulatory Process

The regulatory process is lengthy and fairly complicated. Recently there has been much interest expressed in it often from a critical standpoint since many well-informed individuals both within the industry and outside are of the opinion that the current level of regulatory activity, which is perceived as excessive, is in the process of stifling innovatory activity altogether. Many papers have been produced to indicate that the development time of pharmaceutical products is ever-lengthening. It might be said that this in itself is no bad thing. However, it does appear that the lengthening timescale for development does not necessarily confer additional benefits in terms of product safety when the pharmaceutical is eventually released for use in man.

Regulatory activity in some countries is more highly developed than in others. Consequently those territories which have developed a lengthy and complicated regulatory process often tend to admit pharmaceutical products to the market much later than those where regulations are less stringent. One such country is the USA and the Food and Drug Administration has, in the past, been held to be responsible for a 'drug lag' between the USA and other economically developed, but slightly less stringently regulated, countries. Of course the protagonists of regulatory activity argue that this drug lag has in fact prevented the USA from experiencing some of the untoward effects associated with some modern pharmaceutical innovations. Notable among these is Practolol, which reached the market in the UK some time before it even became registrable in the USA. The time lag was sufficient to allow the untoward effects in the UK to show up, with the result that the registration process in the USA could be stopped. Damage from this particular pharmaceutical to large numbers of the population of the USA was therefore prevented. On the other hand, it must be stated that a large number of people who could otherwise have benefited significantly from Practolol therapy never had the opportunity to do so.

If the regulatory process is long and complicated and leads to large numbers of individuals not having the opportunity to benefit from new medicines, the question 'Why have the regulatory process at all?' might be asked, and as a corollary of this, 'How did it get so lengthy and complicated?'

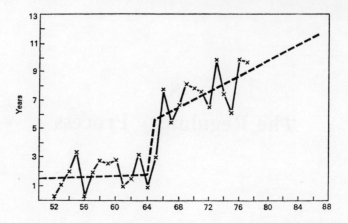

Figure 40 Showing the significant increase in the time lag between first publication and marketing, which accelerated about 1964 and has been increasing since. (Redrawn from Cromie, in *Medicines for the Year 2000*.)

ORIGINS OF REGULATIONS

Originally regulations were introduced in various countries to prevent adulteration of standard remedies and to circumvent unscrupulous individuals swindling the public by peddling quack medicines. The original objective therefore was to ensure quality of the stated article. That is, that the product did indeed contain what was stated on the label, and therefore the public knew when they were buying the medicine that they were getting what they were paying for. Another reason for regulations of a slightly different kind operated with respect to drugs which were perceived as liable to produce a problem of addiction or abuse. The regulations also governed the manufacture, sale and supply of such medicines.

These fairly rudimentary regulations were in operation for a long period of time in a number of different territories. Meanwhile pharmaceutical science advanced and medicines of increasing degrees of sophistication were produced. As nearly everyone is aware, the Thalidomide tragedy occurred with the result that the ensuing public outcry demanded that governments acted to ensure that medicines were reasonably safe for their intended use. Consequently the regulatory process had advanced along the road from 'quality assurance' to a demand for safety. This advance occurred at different rates in different countries, but in general the result was that various changes were established which sought to guarantee, as far as the science of the day could ensure it, that the intended new medicine had been properly tested and that the regulations had been applied to both pre-clinical and clinical investigations.

Eventually it came to be realised that certain medicines were of dubious efficacy, and that while they might be pre-eminently safe, it could not be stated that they were positively aiding the patient. With the accent principally on the clinical area of testing, regulatory advances moved along the pathway slowly and surely of demanding efficacy data, i.e. proof that the new pharmaceutical would actually benefit the conditions which it was intended to treat. By the end of the 1970s the regulatory process had steadily advanced along the road to the extent where proof of quality, safety and efficacy was required.

Currently however, matters are in the process of advancing yet further, since a number of pharmaceutical companies naturally working in the same areas of interest have produced pharmaceuticals which have broadly similar actions and activities. As described above, this often arises because either certain disease areas have larger populations than others and are therefore more profitable, or because of the current status of animal testing procedures where the most reliable pharmacological predictive results are generated in these areas. This has led to a large number of compounds in certain areas which all have a broadly similar therapeutic activity. Because they do have this broadly similar activity, certain sovereign regulatory agencies, in an effort to contain the costs of their health services, have (informally at any rate) introduced a fourth major requirement into their regulatory or pharmaceutical licensing activity – that of utility.

This constant march of regulatory activity has meant that fewer and fewer pharmaceuticals actually reach the market since it is obvious that the more stringent the regulations, the more difficult it is to satisfy them. In addition larger amounts of any R & D budget are taken up in applying the various testing procedures demanded, and since money supply is in every situation finite, less and less is available for innovatory research. Certainly viewing recent statistical, analytical and computer models it might be postulated that if the process is allowed to continue at its current rate medical innovations could cease before the year 2000 since it would be impossible to provide the funds to develop them to the degree required. This ever-lengthening development pathway has yet another important effect, which is that a company will normally seek to patent its discovery as soon as it believes it has something worth protecting. With a long development process, it follows that the earlier it applies for this patent the shorter will be the period for exclusivity to market at the end. This will naturally affect views on the financial return of the discovery no matter how important it is. Currently in the UK, patent life is of the order of twenty years; whereas in the late 1960s and early 1970s when it took only three or four years to develop a new pharmaceutical speciality, a company could expect, say, twelve years of exclusivity to exploit their discovery (at that time patent life was sixteen years). Now, however, if the development pathway takes twelve years, the company, with an extension from sixteen to twenty years of patent life, can only expect eight years of exclusivity, and so on. It can be readily seen that if development takes fifteen or sixteen years for a particularly difficult compound (and often true innovations are difficult since new ground is continually being broken) it may be that the four or five years remaining for exclusive exploitation is too short for the company to even recoup its expenditure over the last fifteen or sixteen years, let alone make a profit. Such a milieu would be bound to affect investment and therefore drug innovation.

REGULATORY AFFAIRS IN THE PHARMACEUTICAL INDUSTRY

As government agencies established regulatory bodies, so also did the specialty of Regulatory Officer arise within the pharmaceutical industry, and regulatory departments were developed wherein reposed detailed information on the regulations in various countries and which provided the working interface between the government and the company. The regulatory function within a pharmaceutical company has a most important duty to discharge. Basically it is responsible for ensuring that when a regulatory submission is made to a government, compliance of data exists as required by the law in that territory. The function is also responsible for ensuring that the quality of data are appropriate, that the information used is clear and concise and that the conclusions drawn from the experiments are a fair representation of what was actually performed and what the results were. Specialists within the regulatory function therefore must have the appropriate scientific knowledge to enable them to interpret correctly what the dossier contains. They are also responsible for ensuring that the arrangement of the data is satisfactory so that all major conclusions are easily traceable to original material and that the overall physical quality of the dossier is of an appropriate standard.

It follows therefore that the regulatory function is involved in the drug development process right from the start since many of the reports which will be used in the final submitted dossier will be written perhaps five or six years or more before they are used. Of course, considering this period of time, various national regulations may be changed. Again it is the responsibility of the regulatory function to ensure that reports generated even some years earlier remain valid.

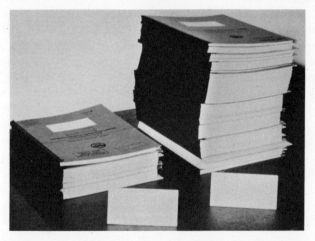

Figure 41   Illustrating the continual increase in data required by regulatory authorities. The three broadly comparable submissions show data required in 1972, 1978 and 1980, respectively.

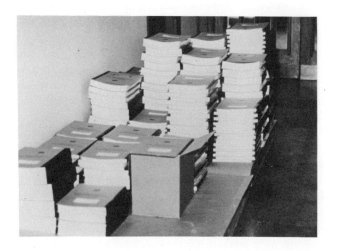

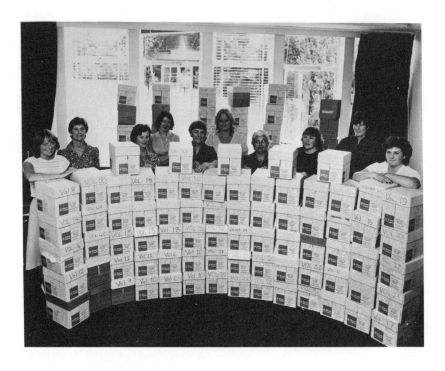

Figure 41 (continued)

REGULATORY AFFAIRS INTERACTIONS

Apart from the interactive on-going relationship a regulatory affairs department will have with government drug registration agencies, the first major point of formal contact will be when the company applies to proceed from the pre-clinical to the clinical phase. In many territories the data thus far generated have to be submitted together with the company's proposals for the next phase - the clinical studies. When this data and the proposals have been examined and found to be appropriate the company gains a Clinical Trial 'Certificate' or permission to proceed. Sometimes this is done 'by default' as in the USA, where if the company does not hear from the Food and Drug Administration within thirty days to the contrary, it can proceed. During this clinical phase, however, the closest liaison is maintained between the company and the government agency so that the latter is kept fully informed of the progress of the programme.

Eventually, when a company considers that it has sufficient knowledge about a new compound to enable it to apply to a national regulatory body for a licence to market it, all of the data which has been collected and collated together are assembled into a dossier representing the sum total of the company's knowledge about its new medicine. This will extend from the early stages involving detailed descriptions of the manufacture of the basic chemical, together with all the detailed information on its basic scientific characteristics, e.g. quality and will then lead on to a full description of the various animal studies which have been done over different timescales and which when taken together give some indication of safety. The third major portion, with its roots in animal pharmacology, leading through human pharmacology and into the clinical studies, will seek to indicate that efficacy is proven. Of course, the actual order of 'chapters' in the submitted dossier will vary from territory to territory although all will require detailed explanation to enable them to evaluate that the above criteria of quality, safety and efficacy have now been met. Neither absolute safety nor, indeed, absolute efficacy, can be guaranteed in each individual. The dossier therefore will be directed towards assessing accurately the risk–benefit ratio and in what particular patient population this is most advantageous.

HARMONISATION OF REGULATIONS

If the development pathway is a long one leading to erosion of patent life, successful companies will try to obtain registration in a wide number of territories at or about the same time, since by this process it will hope to maximise the return on investment. In some areas of the world there have been attempts over the last few years to harmonise regulations in such a way that when these supra-national regulations have been satisfied, the company is empowered to sell its new product in a whole series of similarly developed territories. Such harmonisation is tending to occur where economic union already exists. Two ready examples are the harmonisation within the EEC and a certain degree of uniformity within the Scandinavian group of countries. At the end of this stage of development the company concerned, having accumulated all this knowledge about its new pharmacological product, will be in a position to advise the medical profession directly on how much of the product is to be used, in which patients, over which particular period of time, and indeed what benefit the doctor can reasonably expect by so doing. At the same time that the registration dossier is submitted it will be accompanied by a complete direction circular to the physician which will summarise accurately all the information gained up until that time. This direction circular will make claims for the product's efficacy and will delineate the risk. In effect it is the job of the government regulatory agency to examine the dossier when it is submitted to them in order to ascertain that the claims made for the new product are substantiated and that the degree of risk is as stated.

SUBMISSION OF THE DOSSIER

The dossier having been compiled is therefore submitted to various national regulatory agencies which have the unenviable task of being sited between the pharmaceutical industry (applicant) and the medical profession and patients (indirect and direct consumers). This might be perceived as being reasonably simple in itself. However, because of the involvement of the public as a consumer, regulatory authorities are subject to all the problems and pressures generated by minority groups, the media and politicians. If they approve a medicine quickly and it turns out later to have deleterious effects in a significant number of patients they will be pilloried for either not assessing the dossier properly or for being too hasty in approving it. On the other hand, if they delay unduly in some territories they could be accused of increasing human suffering and perhaps even contributing to mortality figures by such a delay. Because of the uncertainty of (and indeed the perceived importance of) *guaranteeing absolute safety*, new requirements and regulations are constantly being added to the already existing plethora. This means in effect that the regulatory agency is tending to delay the decision and indeed a dossier can be with some regulatory agencies for four years or more before a decision, either positive or negative, is received by the company.

Since it is widely accepted that animal tests and indeed clinical studies to the degree and extent required for a product licence application will not necessarily indicate the true risk–benefit ratio of a new compound, moves are currently afoot to shorten the timescale towards formal licence approval of a new medicine (which may have to be revoked if untoward effects manifest themselves) by various forms of monitored release. The reasons for this and the methods employed will be more fully described in later chapters.

As we have seen, in many territories the relationship with a government agency does not commence with the submission of the dossier requesting permission to market the compound. It begins in fact with a request of varying degrees of formality to commence clinical studies. The animal evidence generated up until that time is presented so that the company may be allowed to proceed to clinical testing. The protocols for such clinical studies are submitted and approved by the regulatory agency at that time. Because of the large number of new pharmaceutical specialties requiring approval in this way, this system produced a delay in many countries which was largely considered unacceptable, because at that stage the company did not know whether it had anything of therapeutic value or not. Building on FDA experience, recently a system of exemption has been adopted in some territories whereby when the information is submitted a definitive period of time is allowed to elapse, after which if the government regulatory agency has either not responded or requested an extension, the company may proceed to clinical testing.

EARLIER HUMAN EXPERIENCE

Overall, the current movements in this vexed arena are towards more early introduction to man in selected, carefully monitored and controlled patient populations with continuous interpretation of the results and a commitment on the part of the company to hold or suspend the programme should anything untoward occur. This has the beneficial effect of allowing companies with products of marginal efficacy or of dubious safety immediately to limit the extent of their investment. In an ideal world this is how it would be, but in practical terms because of international differences between regulatory bodies and requirements together with different responses in dissimilar populations, a significant amount of international investment is still required.

DIALOGUE

Undoubtedly, together with various exemption procedures, the way forward consists of effective dialogue between companies and regulatory agencies in the first instance involving mainly those who are responsible for compiling the dossier, but also those who have actually generated the work, having been in constant and close contact. Therefore problems can be effectively answered as and when they arise and the overall approval process very much facilitated. It cannot be too strongly emphasised that there is no such thing as absolute safety and efficacy and that no one individual or group of individuals is necessarily paramount in accurately judgeing and interpreting data from both pre-clinical and clinical experiments which are continually breaking new ground.

QUALITY ASSURANCE OF DATA

Finally, although more will be said later about computerisation statistics and information science (which are also interlocked with regulatory affairs), mention must be made of a function the existence of which has already been implied.

This is quality assurance of all data which a company submits to a licensing authority. In these days of long laborious regulatory processes it is perhaps understandable, but not forgivable, that occasional forged laboratory notebooks and falsified patient record forms make their appearance. This quality assurance function of all regulatory affairs departments is time consuming but all important, not only from an internal standpoint but also from an external standpoint, since the validity of general and research management decisions to progress or abandon a project may well depend on it. Additionally, for the public to be put at possible risk through misleading data, is clearly unacceptable.

9
Marketing

MARKETING

Although in some research establishments the concept of marketing input and involvement may not be a popular notion, good marketing technique is essential to the full and successful exploitation of any product, including pharmaceuticals. Conversely it is probably true to say that not even the best marketing function can 'make a silk purse out of a sow's ear'. A commercial success, on a sustained basis at any rate, cannot be achieved with a medicine offering little in the way of benefit, no matter how intense are the efforts of a very professional and competent marketing department.

Obviously there are degrees of achievement between these two extremes and it has been mentioned earlier that to increase the eventual chances of success the aim must be to involve marketing people at the earliest stages of the research and development process. Doing so brings a number of benefits. Firstly, it gains commitment from marketing personnel towards the product candidates the company is developing or hoping to develop. Secondly, it provides a forum for the cross-fertilisation of ideas – R & D does not have a monopoly on ideas and those coming from individuals standing just a little way back from the immediate problem can often usefully throw light on the way ahead. Thirdly, it commences the process of educational familiarisation at the embryonal stage. Because the marketing function through its medical representatives will provide the final pathway in the presentation of the pharmaceutical company's products to its public (i.e. the medical profession), this concept of early familiarisation by marketing personnel is crucial. So much so that it cannot really start early enough. Especially so since the product mix and product type embodies the whole ethos of the company. Commitment from marketing to the company's present and future products can only be created in any lasting form by this educative familiarisation. It is essential for maximum success, particularly in the light of the necessity for international marketing to succeed.

For long the Cinderella of many pharmaceutical companies, the marketing departments of the vast majority are now mature and responsible organisations that participate fully and constructively in the progress from chemical to new medicine. Apart from the perhaps obvious benefit of preventing R & D from developing a product the marketing department does not wish to sell (and this has happened in the past), the closeness of co-operation directly aids the company as a whole since the process of planning for eventual product introductions is better thought out and therefore more objective. No pharmaceutical company operates in isolation and consequently must be constantly aware of changing market forces and the new product developments of other companies. This is necessary to ensure that a new medicine is introduced at the most opportune time. This has now become an international, rather than a national, consideration. Since any introduction of a new product in one or a number of different territories costs a considerable amount of money, it has an important bearing on company cash-flow. Therefore the timing of each new product introduction and where it will be introduced can be critical to the success of the whole operation.

By a gradual process of enlightenment the 'ivory towers' of R & D have been opened up to outside scrutiny not only by marketing departments but also by other disciplines. In general this has been advantageous from the combined standpoints of the public at large, the company and those departments directly involved.

PRODUCT MANAGEMENT

More will be said in the next chapter about *project* management, which is probably the current Cinderella within pharmaceutical product development, but at this stage it must be mentioned if only to heighten awareness of the interlocking of this new discipline with marketing. Marketing is now an extremely specialised business and pharmaceuticals are no exception. The expertise and knowledge required to market a cardiovascular product successfully are different in many major respects from those skills required to market and sell antibiotics. The same is true of other product categories. In view of this a system of *product* management has evolved whereby the product specialist (manager) is involved with the progress of his product long before it comes to a marketable stage. To do this he works closely with his more scientifically orientated counterpart, a project manager who has been responsible (see later) for piloting his 'baby' from the embryonic stages of early R & D. This is where the process of familiarisation or education starts. It is like osmosis since the product (and project) manager 'absorbs' much of his knowledge almost unconsciously during detailed discussions with toxicologists, pharmacologists, physicians and scientists from other disciplines, such as formulation development.

PRODUCT IDENTITY

Contact with this latter discipline (i.e. formulation development) is very important since the eventual evolution of a discernible product identity will depend upon it to a significant degree. The product manager, in consultation both with his colleagues in the marketing department and those in external specialised agencies, will have been conducting early research into the perceived deficiencies of presently available therapy. Perhaps it consists of tablets which are too large and difficult to swallow, or the tablets have to be taken too many times a day, or even that the tablets are packaged in such a way that they are difficult to get at. These are only a few representative reasons – the list can be almost endless. Some are more important than others, but in any event they may serve to focus attention on this precept of early marketing involvement since clearly there is little sense in R & D producing a large clumsy tablet which the patients cannot easily swallow, or developing a medicine to be taken three times a day when patients will not take a midday dose, even that the tablets are packaged in a bottle which patients with severe rheumatoid arthritis cannot open. The above examples are perhaps simplistic but should serve to illustrate that the progress of many an effective medicine has been slowed or even jeopardised in the past because these seemingly minor points were not adequately considered. On a more major scale, detailed research may indicate that a certain proportion of the patient population is being inadequately treated or that their condition is not being controlled. All of these aspects of development, both major and minor, have to be carefully built up over a period of time.

Different marketing departments have particular areas of expertise and also likes and dislikes, just like anyone else. Consequently, they may consider that they are better at presenting or selling tablets rather than suspensions or capsules. Alternatively, they may prefer particular forms of unit dosage, e.g. blister packing as opposed to foil wrapping. These considerations too have to be programmed early into development because the appropriate dosage form and its packaging will have to be prepared, tried and tested long before registration of the product is even applied for. Therefore involvement and communication between marketing departments and various development disciplines can save that most important element in a product's life – time.

MARKET RESEARCH

The liaison between a marketing department and various specialised external (to the company) agencies has been commented upon briefly. While development is proceeding, the marketing department will commission various elements of market research from these agencies by which it is hoped to identify the major dynamics of the particular market that the new product will enter. At or about this time, the marketing department, in consultation with the medical department in charge of the clinical research and the external agency, will initiate the identification of a product profile. Since this occurs in the development process well before registration it is unlikely that the marketing department will have definitive answers to all of its questions. Perhaps if events continued without modification, a number of important (to a marketing department) will have definitive answers to all of its questions. Perhaps if events continued without modification, a number of important (to a marketing department) questions might still remain unanswered at the end of the development process. Consequently, the clinical trial programme might conceivably be modified or augmented so that answers to these various questions can be obtained. Another way of attempting to answer questions in order to define accurately a new medicine's profile is for both marketing and agency personnel to talk directly to many of the practising physicians who have participated in the clinical trial programme.

ADVERTISING DEVELOPMENT

As this process continues, both the marketing department and the outside agency it has briefed to help it, will be building up a concept of the product which will extend into various pieces of illustrative matter together with printed copy. Thus the advertising campaign is born. This has now to be tested on a panel of doctors to ensure that the message it is desired to transmit is actually being received clearly and unequivocally. The various advertisements must conform to an industry-wide code of practice both for general format and subject matter (for instance, they must not be of a sexually suggestive nature, tasteless or misleading from a technical standpoint), and they must of course be scientifically accurate. This latter criterion is ensured by checks both within the company (by its medical department) and by the regulatory agency, since all scientifically informative material (such as data sheets, etc) has to be submitted to government agencies for their approval.

SALES TRAINING

Therefore before a company actually gains registration for its new product, the marketing department has been working on it for some considerable time but always in anticipation of its eventual successful registration by various national authorities. Eventually, news of the expected product will have filtered down to the various forces of medical representatives within the company. But not to each and every sales force at the beginning, since the company will have a number of prime territories where it will initially launch the new medicine. This will give the company the best chance of success because effort will be concentrated. However, when appropriate, the educative process will be invoked so that the medical representatives will start to absorb the salient features of the physiology and pathology of the condition or conditions in the area of therapy that the new medicine will be entering. They will be given a concept of the disease area together with a history of the development of therapy for that particular thera-peutic problem. Having painted the background, the training team will then indicate how they see the new medicine fitting in. Sales training will then begin in earnest because by this time the new product is either registered or very close to it, and the launch dates in a small group of critical territories will have been established. Furthermore, the representatives' help may need to be enlisted in conducting an additional clinical trial involving perhaps thousands of patients. This will use a fairly simple trial protocol, the aim of which is to provide the company with more definitive information on efficacy and side-effects which may not have been possible hitherto because of the finite resources of the medical department. This is a pre-marketing utilisation trial. However, this device, though a useful one in research terms, must not be used as a method to 'buy prescriptions' from 'day one' after launch, but it can yield much useful market intelligence on doctors' prescribing and usage patterns and doctor–patient attitudes. It can gauge the effectiveness of the marketing 'story' and so aid in defining the niche for the new product. Before being able to present effectively the new medicine to the medical profession, medical representatives therefore have to be trained specifically with regard to its character and utilisation including the overall context in which it will be used. Many disciplines within the pharmaceutical company will be united in this training aspect through a system of formal lectures and seminars. An increasingly high degree of professionalism is now being demanded from medical representatives and this means that they have to be familiar with the new product's main actions and advantages and also to have a realistic and balanced view of its disadvantages. This sales training is very important since the medical representative is the 'final pathway' between a company and its public, i.e. the medical profession. Medical representatives have a key role in informing the physician about a new product, and during that product's life in keeping him up to date on its usage and progress.

INFORMATION FLOW

At the same time that medical representatives exercise this essential function of informing physicians about new therapeutic developments, they also fulfil the converse responsibility. That is, they will receive information from the medical profession on the relative performance of the new medicine both in a variety of different patient types and also versus the competition. It may be that, despite long involvement with the product, careful product planning and a seemingly effective product introduction, the new medicine is not being used as widely as the company had hoped. It appears that the company has 'got it wrong'. In attempting to 'get it right' and in order to get at the truth, the company will rely to an extent on feedback from prescribing physicians either spontaneously or by questionnaire, or by direct contact with the medical representative or company medical-department staff. There may be a number of significant pointers, such as either inappropriate dosage or selection of the wrong patients, which will need to be checked out using a more formal type of approach, such as a post-marketing utilisation trial. On the other hand, the advertising campaign may have simply failed to 'get through'. Whatever the reason, it will need to be identified and corrected either intercurrently or, in some instances, by a complete relaunch of the product.

Certain information of a critical nature from another standpoint may also be generated informally. Many first indications of severely deleterious side-effects are often received in this way. What happens is that a physician meeting a company's medical representative for perhaps only a very short period of time alerts that representative to the existence of an unexplained and untoward effect when that particular physician prescribed the medicine. This information, properly transmitted and then co-ordinated through the company's main office, can serve as an extremely sensitive early-warning system with regard to the possible existence of unsuspected severe adverse effects. Of course, once notified of such an effect, the company has a duty to follow it up and also to inform the National Registration Agency — more will be said about this aspect of development in a later chapter.

From a different standpoint this contact between physician and representative can be extremely beneficial. The latter receives physicians' impressions and observations following usage of the new medicine and this may facilitate the identification of new patient groups who would benefit from the medication. In addition, it may contribute signally to the development of subsequent indications which might be commercially more significant than the one which was first developed. This particular aspect of product life is an important one and will be examined in more detail below.

BASIC INFORMATION: INVESTIGATORS' BROCHURE TO PRODUCT MONOGRAPH

Although not specifically mentioned in the clinical section, the production of a creditable and regularly updated (clinical) investigators' brochure which contains a summary of the animal and clinical work on which the product profile is based, is an important step. Important not only as a working document for those actively engaged in clinical research, but also as a base document from which many of the marketing department's promotional elements will be derived. Most marketing departments will produce a marketing base document from this investigators' brochure, and afterwards, in tandem with the specialised external marketing agency, build up a series of folders for the representative to use during discussions with the doctor, materials for mailings and formal advertisements. Of course, like other areas of development, this process starts off fairly simply and indeed speculatively, but as knowledge builds up it becomes increasingly more objective and sophisticated. By the time that registration is being applied for in a number of major territories, an authoritative product monograph will be in existence which can then be used as a basis for all future marketing activities. With a dynamic product it will never be a truly definitive document because knowledge is continually accumulating and being added, but its 'rate of change' will slow down as the product becomes established. In any event, this document and many others within a pharmaceutical company will be assiduously updated at established intervals in order to ensure its constant accuracy.

Therefore, the marketing department's input throughout all stages of the development process is critical to the success or failure of the new medicine. Their gradual assimilation of knowledge over the years that the compound has been undergoing development will be extremely important, not only at the launch conference but also beyond. If they know the product well and believe in its capabilities they will transmit this with confidence and enthusiasm to their medical representative sales forces, who will then present the product efficiently to the medical profession. As noted at the beginning of this chapter, 'it is impossible to make a silk purse out of a sow's ear', either by slick marketing techniques or by unjustified claims for a significant period of time, and a product which does not live up to the profession's expectations will simply not be commercially viable.

10
Project Co-ordination

By sharing in the universal problem, all pharmaceutical companies compete for resources. Thankfully there always seem to be more ideas than there are funds to carry them out, but this brings its own problems. Particularly over the last decade, the development process has become extended. It is now much more complex and correspondingly more costly. Some of this increase, both in time and cost, can be directly attributable to increased regulatory activity. There are not only delays produced by the need to satisfy greatly increased requirements under the enacted legislation and its regulations, but also those delays introduced through the time it takes a regulatory agency to assimilate the information it has asked for (and been presented with) and come to a decision – four years in some instances. However, the time taken to generate and obtain products has also been increased because much more time and effort now has to be spent on the devising and evaluation of basic scientific methodologies. Increasing amounts of basic research now have to be done to produce each product opportunity. Consequently, for any company to succeed with R & D, the number of projects it can operate at any given time has necessarily to be restricted. It is the responsibility of the research director, or other senior operating manager, in consultation with his commercial and financial colleagues, to assess the projects in the company's portfolio and to determine which will offer the best financial return to the company within an optimum timescale. Probably one of the most difficult and important decisions to be taken by such a group is when to stop a project, because a project which apparently cannot succeed in any reasonable timescale will utilise resources which could be more properly and effectively allocated elsewhere. And it has been said that for every project terminated just short of success, there are probably a hundred more which go on for too long. Be that as it may, it is always difficult to stop a project if only for the reason that dedicated specialists with a passionate belief in their particular work are involved. It is not easy to redeploy such individuals precipitously, and it is probably best done by gentle changes in emphasis and direction rather than by sudden sideways or about-face turns. This means that projects will tend to 'wither away' rather than suddenly cease like turning off a tap.

Some projects will necessarily be longer term than others and most companies strive to achieve a balance between short-term projects which might produce a moderate revenue and those longer-term ventures which, if successful, could revolutionise the practice of medicine and produce relatively large cash returns. Obviously such ventures are risky not only from the point of view of the many pitfalls along the development pathway (animal toxicity, lack of clinical efficacy or a rare but serious unwanted effect), but also the risk of being pipped at the post by a competitor.

PROJECT MANAGEMENT

It is in an effort to ensure that *all* projects proceed at an optimum rate and that all unnecessary time lapses are removed from the system that project management has evolved. The project manager may be responsible for just one or a number of projects, depending on their complexity. His job is essentially to ensure that projects do not 'get in each other's way' by competing simultaneously for scarce resources within the R & D establishment. Since the project manager operates outside the disciplines of the line departments, he must have good inter-personal skills and be sufficiently aware of all the various scientific disciplines so that he can appreciate the obligatory timescales involved. At the same time he must not fall prey to the occasional prima donna who is striving for absolute perfection in his particular part of the project, which might unjustifiably hold up everything. The project system therefore operates, as a type of matrix, functionally across the line departments. It acts as a lubricant in the interstices of the total R & D effort, but always with the objective that the needs of the priority projects are paramount.

CRITICAL PATHS

How, then, is this objective fulfilled? In its simplest form the progress of any project is monitored by means of a written-down critical-path analysis. The various steps or activities necessary to develop the new medicine are all listed down the left-hand side of a large piece of paper and against a linear scale the time anticipated to commence, run and complete each activity is defined on a bar chart. From this bar chart is constructed the critical pathway of development. For a variety of reasons some activities cannot start until others finish (for instance, there must be an adequate supply of pure chemical substance before chronic toxicity, carcinogenicity or large-scale clinical studies can commence). Critical-path analysis allows identification of these interdependent areas and maps out how delay in one discipline might affect progress in another, or indeed how it might affect the whole programme. The analysis is helpful to all in development line-management because it pinpoints when great demands can and will occur in their resources. These can then be suitably planned for (e.g. the ordering of adequate numbers of animals for a test and the provision of

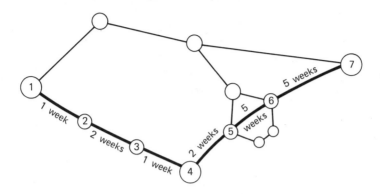

Figure 42 A very simple activity diagram together with a critical path. If any of the activities on the 'loops' takes longer than that allowed for on the critical path, it may need to be revised, since the timing of the whole project could be thrown out of synchrony. Of course the critical pathway and activity diagram for the total drug development process is bewilderingly complicated.

suitable facilities to house them). Such planning should minimise delays because it identifies likely problems before they arise.

One critical path for one project can be complicated enough. When this is repeated, say, twenty times and all of these projects are running concurrently but at different rates (since they will have started at different times and have different degrees of priority), it can be readily appreciated how complex the whole operation is. For this reason project management is a discipline in itself and is complicated enough to require computer input if three or four important projects are not all going to be competing for the same vital resources simultaneously. If this were to happen it would be clearly counter-productive. The project manager, as a co-ordinator *par excellence*, has the primary aim of ensuring that such resource competition is identified to research management so that a decision can be taken, after having involved all interested parties, on which programme or project will have priority. Because there is always competition for resources it is readily apparent that effective project management and co-ordination is vital for the success of development in any company.

11
Manufacture and Supply

So far very little mention has been made of this highly critical area. The chemical invented on the chemist's bench, often in minute quantities, and its analysis and characteristics, have already been described. Proceeding onwards, the next step is the chemical development laboratory where the chemical synthesis becomes fully established and a pilot batch is manufactured.

Usually, by the time it has been proved that the synthesis 'works' on a large scale and produces material to an acceptable degree of purity, the overall development programme is far advanced in other areas. Provided there is sufficient chemical to satisfy the requirements of the animal (pharmacology and toxicology) pharmaceutical formulation and clinical studies, it is usual to delay definitive work on the chemical plant until (using critical-path analysis) the registration application dates and possible launch dates have become more positive. Once a launch date is set even tentatively the production department will have to draw up its own critical path to ensure that it can build, commission and 'de-bug' a chemical plant to produce the active pure chemical in suitable quantities at the required time. Of course, the amounts actually required will vary depending upon the clinical dosage of the compound. Therefore a potent agent used at a dosage of 0.3 mg will yield more than 300 doses per gram, whereas a different agent normally used in 500 mg doses will yield only two doses per gram. Ignoring possible differences in the length and complexity of the chemical synthesis involved, the first substance could probably be made in a relatively small laboratory using equipment costing of the order of a few thousand pounds, whereas the other chemical (500 mg dose) might require a vast cehmical complex occupying several acres and costing of the order of a few million pounds. In the latter example, the later the decision to commit can be taken the better for the company's cash flow. On the other hand, it must not be so late that the whole launch of what might possibly be a significant therapeutic advance is put in jeopardy because the commissioning programme runs into unforeseen snags. It is a delicate balancing act.

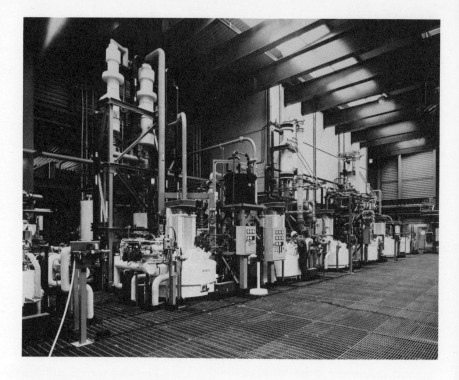

Figure 43   A modern pharmaceutical chemical production facility.

SUPPLY OF PURE CHEMICAL

The major responsibility of the production department is therefore to ensure an
adequate supply of the pure active chemical. It achieves this by scaling up the
synthesis, if necessary, from kilograms to perhaps thousands of tonnes. Through
liaison with the R & D department it builds on the experience and knowledge
gained in the chemical development laboratory where a more limited scale-up
has already been effected.

FORMULATION SCALE-UP

Similarly (and often concurrently) the production department is involved in
another scale-up operation. It must take the formulation developed by the
pharmacists in the formulation development department and commence procedures to ensure that the formulation (whatever it is — tablets, capsules, gels,
injections, etc) will 'run' on a large scale. There may be a problem here since it
may not be possible to do this until sufficiently large quantities of chemical have
been made. If it is a question of delaying the capital investment, then usually
this interim supply of up to perhaps a tonne of pure chemical, is put out to

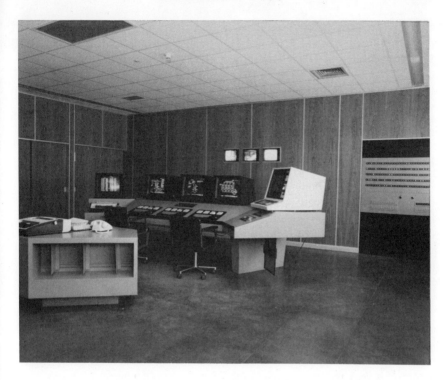

Figure 44 A computerised production control room.

contract manufacture. Close monitoring of the problems encountered by the contract manufacturer by the commissioning company often pays dividends since snags which are encountered in producing a tonne can be identified and overcome. This knowledge can then be used when the company itself takes over the production of the chemical.

Often a formulation which is perfectly satisfactory when operated on relatively small-scale pilot-plant machinery by formulation development scientists will not perform satisfactorily in larger batches. The formulation, and perhaps even the procedure, may require to be modified, sometimes extensively, before the problems are resolved. Depending upon the modifications actually carried out, it may in turn be necessary to perform additional clinical (bioequivalence) work (see later) to show that the new formulation behaves clinically in a directly comparable way to the old one. The degree of scale-up may require the production of thousands of tablets an hour to satisfy the anticipated demand. If the product is to be a tablet, appropriate sets of suitably designed punches must be ordered in good time for the production machines. Similarly, additional equipment may be needed to produce other formulations.

As early as possible in the development process, samples of the tablets, capsules, gel, etc will have been packaged and put into storage for the stability-testing procedures already described. If the formulation is then changed for production reasons later on this early work will be invalidated. It must therefore be repeated using the then final formulation in the final packaging. These and other examples serve to illustrate the importance of the principle (which cannot be overstressed) of getting the pure chemical specification and the formulation specification settled as early as possible in development because it is the foundation of all later work. Changes inevitably cause delays and delays cost money.

PACK DEVELOPMENT AND SCALE-UP

Another area of transition from the laboratory to factory is that of pack development. As elsewhere, a significant amount of co-ordination is required here between the pack development laboratory, marketing department and the factory personnel. As perhaps a ludicrous example, it is clearly counterproductive if the pack development laboratory establishes a stable formulation in glass bottles when the marketing department wants a 'blister'-type pack and the factory is geared up with machinery to handle metal-foil wrapping. The coordination input from the project manager aided by the product manager from the marketing department should prevent such a set of circumstances from arising. It will alert the production department to the need to order, if not already in their possession, appropriate machinery to satisfy the need. If new machinery is necessary, it must be commissioned and run in order to 'de-bug' it before it is required to manufacture launch stocks. Of course, it almost goes without saying that adequate stocks of the new medicine (and suitably packaged) must be available well in advance of the anticipated launch so that they can be efficiently distributed to the various wholesalers' warehouses. Not too far in advance though, because tying up money in this way for longer than is strictly necessary might constrain another area of the business.

GOOD MANUFACTURING PRACTICE

Just because possibly millions of tablets, thousands of bottles and hundreds or even thousands of injections are produced in a pharmaceutical factory every week is no reason for it to be untidy, dirty or badly organised. Under the various national food-and-drugs or medicines acts provisions are made to inspect factory premises at regular intervals and to compare their activities with various procedural rules under those acts. These good-manufacturing practices are established procedures and must be observed if the company is to maintain its licence to manufacture pharmaceuticals in that territory.

The purpose of the various good-manufacturing-practice regulations is to ensure that raw materials coming into the factory are indeed what they are claimed to be and that they are not contaminated by insects, rodents, birds or other extraneous animal life, nor should they be exposed to the elements. The same is true of partially processed materials and finished goods. Because every pharmaceutical production plant deals with a number of different products, there must be stringent methods written down, understood and observed by every employee to ensure that 'cross contamination' of products cannot occur. This is achieved by dividing production into distinct lines which produce finished goods in defined batches. Great emphasis is placed on batch identity whatever the stage of production so that an identifiable quantity of pure active chemical is mixed with identifiable quantities of excipients and then (for instance) tableted and packaged as one lot. Thus if anything untoward is suspected later with any of the boxes of tablets from that batch the whereabouts of *all* the boxes from that batch can be identified, and, if necessary, recalled to the factory by well-organised recall procedures. The history and progress of the materials including their quality checks along the production line can be fully established through the documentation created during production. Full investigation of any untoward event is consequently completely possible.

IDENTIFICATION OF BATCHES

Various encoding machines are therefore incorporated in the different lines which are themselves monitored to ensure batch identity and integrity. As production proceeds, small quantities of each batch at different stages of manufacture are withdrawn by scientists working in a quality-control section. It is their function to examine and test all such samples to ensure that they conform to the specifications laid down. By this process the historical documentation is created.

Nowadays pharmaceutical production facilities resemble operating-theatre suites. Often they can be entered only through an airlock where the worker has to change his clothes and perhaps take a shower. Once inside the facility, it is not only well lit but also lined with tile or other material which can be cleaned effectively. As already noted, within the factory, production lines are separate and all the lines are cleared at appropriate intervals. Following this the machinery is subjected to meticulous cleaning. Where necessary, operatives wear gloves to ensure hygiene and if the product demands it (e.g. with hormone production) the operatives are protected from possible deleterious inherent effects (from inhalation) by various dust-control procedures.

The overriding principle in pharmaceutical factory organisation is that there is a 'dirty area' where materials (from chemicals to cardboard packaging) come into the factory. This is separated and distinct from a clean/sterile area where the actual pharmaceuticals are produced. Before leaving this they are usually enclosed in at least two protective coverings. They then travel to a further 'dirty' area where the goods are packaged in outer cartons and await despatch to warehouses. Of course, 'dirty' is only a comparative term since even these parts of the factory are as clean as or cleaner than the average living room.

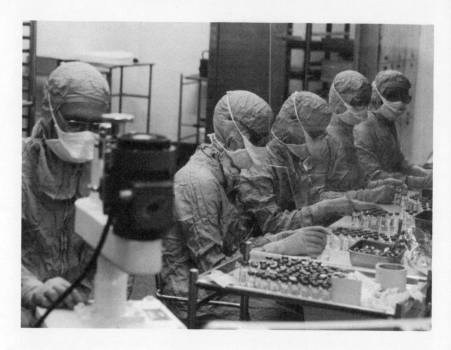

Figure 45   Part of a modern pharmaceutical production area, indicating the high standards of hygiene observed.

The reader can therefore appreciate that the new medicine is produced in a modern factory, safely isolated from other products, in a very clean environment by a batch-type process which is subject to many intricate checks. However, as the recent Tylenol scare indicated, it is more difficult to guarantee the integrity of the product *after* it leaves the factory. But, as subsequent events have shown, it is not impossible since this particular product is now enclosed in elaborate packaging with which it is deemed impossible to tamper without any attempts to do so being immediately apparent. This development serves to reinforce the overriding consideration of all pharmaceutical production activity, which is to ensure the supply of a product of the highest *quality* which is precisely reproducible.

12

The Post-registration Phase

Obviously not even the most efficient company will be able to get simultaneous registration in all the major territories it operates in. However, if well managed and with effective planning it could reasonably expect to get registration in, say, ten territories within a short timescale. Different drug-regulatory authorities have disparate concerns and therefore questions on the submitted dossiers will naturally be different. It will be largely impossible to anticipate the majority of these no matter how perspicacious are the company's regulatory-affairs personnel.

In any event, assuming that the company has registration and has launched the new medicine in, say, 10 major territories, it has therefore entered the post-registration phase. The new medicine will now start to generate money for the company. It will not be making a profit, nor will it do so for some years if the cost of previous research and development (calculated overall since good projects have to fund bad projects) is taken into account.

WIDER EXPOSURE

A number of factors come into play in this post-registration phase. For a start, a number of additional eyes are now on the new medicine. The medical profession has become more widely aware of it. So indeed has the public at large. Politicians and other interested groups will be starting to look at it and measure its performance against the public's expectation of the new treatment and the compound's actual capabilities. Sensationalism is almost inevitable and many people will be awaiting the first signs of toxicity which invariably will be reported. As a result, public confidence in the safety of drug treatment prescribed by doctors has been somewhat eroded, particularly recently. In actual fact, drugs are a great deal safer than the public realises, and many of the company's, the medical profession's and government's efforts will now be directed towards making sure that the risk of an unbalanced view of the medicine's possible harmful effects is minimised. The only way to maintain perspective under these circumstances is for the company to be fully aware of all possible problems itself. As we have seen, in a clinical programme which seeks to bring a new medicine before the regulatory authority and therefore the public within reasonable timescale, only limited patient numbers have been studied. They are mainly, but not exclusively, investigated and monitored for efficacy. The twin issues of both acute (but very rare) and more chronic unwanted effects therefore is inevitably an unexplored one, to an extent. The new medicine will have been marketed with a fairly accurate view having been taken of the possible immediate unwanted side-effects and of their likely severity and frequency of occurrence. The nature and character of the rarer side-effects will not be known, nor indeed will the nature and character of these effects engendered after longer-term usage. Most difficult of all to assess are the chances of side-effects arising perhaps some years after treatment with the new medicine was started. Despite an extensive pre-registration programme many drug-interaction effects will remain to be identified.

POST-MARKETING SURVEILLANCE AND ADVERSE REACTIONS

It is for these reasons that various systems of post-marketing surveillance or adverse-event monitoring have been promulgated. Before examining these different methodologies (all attempting to get at the truth), a definition of what an adverse reaction actually is would be appropriate. The definition proposed by Sir Richard Doll in 1972 is probably still as good today as any which have been suggested since. Doll defined an adverse reaction as 'any event that follows the administration of a drug given in the recommended dose, is attributable to the administration of that drug and is harmful to the recipient, the foetus she carries or, by an effect on the gonads, to the recipient's descendants'.

As already mentioned, there will, of course, have been a number of adverse reactions noted during the clinical studies. Most will be of the acute type, i.e. occurring very shortly after taking the new medication, but a few may give an insight into the types of adverse reaction to be expected after more prolonged treatment with the new agent. For many new types of medication (particularly those intended for chronic usage) it is now virtually a statutory requirement in many territories that at least a hundred patients have been treated for one year before registration is granted. Primarily this requirement is to assess whether the effect of the new drug becomes markedly lessened with time, but it will also indicate what types of reactions can occur with more chronic therapy and also what is their severity and incidence. However, it will have very limited utility from the adverse reaction standpoint since it has been calculated that 3000 patients need to have been studied to give a 95% certainty of detecting reactions occurring at the rate of 0.1% risk. Much rarer events will require 10 000 patients or more, which is a Herculean task in terms of administration alone, to say nothing of the difficulties of integrating the results of such a study. In addition, there is that ever-present consideration − the cost. Nonetheless this must be established since the 1 in 10 000 reaction may be either crippling or fatal. The knowledge that such a reaction can arise is vital, but what is even more important is whether such a reaction could be recognised in the early stages of treat-

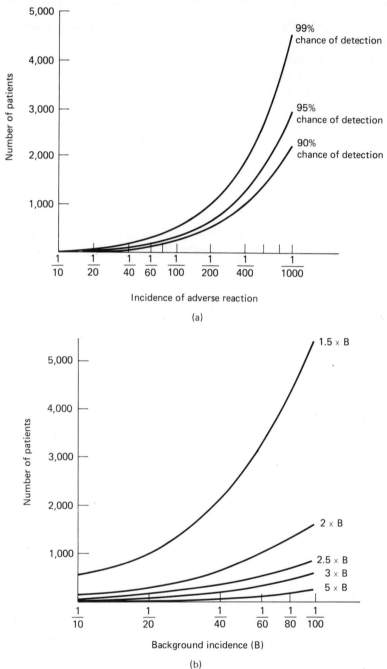

(a)

(b)

Figure 46   Graphs to indicate that to be 99% certain of detecting an adverse reaction arising at a rate of 1 in 1000 some 5000 patients are required. Of course these numbers increase enormously if a background incidence of the particular adverse reaction occurs (b). (Redrawn from Newbould, B. B. in Cavalla, J. F. (1981) (see Bibliography and Suggestions for Further Reading).)

ment, which could then be aborted or modified before such a disastrous outcome ensued.

In the final analysis, efficient adverse-reaction monitoring depends on the attending physician's knowledge and perspicacity, since he alone is probably the only person who knows what the patient is taking and what the course of the patient's condition is likely to be, together with any other details of the case. He is the person ultimately responsible for the totality of management of his patients. Some adverse reactions are expected and indeed are predictable, since they depend directly on the chemical properties of the compound and its clinical pharmacology (e.g. blurred vision, drowsiness and dry mouth observed with certain antihypertensive agents such as alpha-blockers). The vast majority, however, are unfortunately completely unpredictable both from the standpoint of the human pharmacology and also the previous animal pharmacology and toxicology. Herein lies the problem. How can the unforeseen and perhaps unsuspected events be properly identified for what they truly are?

Reporting Methods

For many years various authorities have relied on spontaneous reporting by doctors notifying published or unpublished cases directly to the licensing authority (e.g. the UK's Committee on Safety of Medicines' 'yellow-card' system established in 1963). The results of such reporting are collected, collated and published in tabular form at regular intervals. If a cause for concern appears during the course of the spontaneous reporting then it is drawn to the Committee's attention by those scrutinising the reports if the situation is considered to warrant it. A warning is then transmitted to the prescribing doctors. This system did in fact pick up the Practolol unwanted effect. The only problem lay in the fact that it did not become apparent until five years after the drug was launched. Other methods have relied on intensive monitoring of 'captive' patient groups (either in-patients or out-patients) or epidemiological studies of morbidity and mortality where what medicines the patients took during their last illnesses, etc were also recorded. Large-scale clinical trials have also been employed to the same end.

All approaches have advantages and disadvantages. The majority are relatively cheap to administer but suffer from either great degrees of under-reporting (spontaneous reporting) or delay and difficulty in early recognition of rare, serious, adverse effects. It is the existence of these rare and dramatically life-threatening adverse reactions which creates problems in trying to establish risk-benefit ratio. Therefore with interest focused in this area, different groups or individuals have attempted to create mechanisms which seek to answer this vexed question. These have included various types of post-marketing surveillance. This methodology was behind the introduction of a period of monitored release for a new medicine. Having put forward the view that the release phase should be more tightly controlled, and this having received general acceptance, the question then became one of establishing how it could be done precisely and what were the costs involved.

QUANTITATIVE AND QUALITATIVE SYSTEMS

Post-marketing surveillance may be subdivided into either quantitive systems or qualitative systems. With regard to the former, by restricting release of the new medicine to a limited and known number of physicians (including hospitals, specialists, GPs, etc), the aim was to create a baseline to facilitate the detection of an adverse drug reaction, its incidence and to provide firm evidence of a drug-effect relationship. With a number of different agents going through the system simultaneously it might be possible to produce hard data on *comparative* incidences of effects between drugs. There are a number of drawbacks to such schemes, such as that it introduces a two-tier system of prescribing doctors, it would be expensive (record filling, etc) and would take additional time and work (and therefore cause a problem in obtaining physician co-operation). It would further delay the return to the company of its capital.

Against this, others take the view that the accurate estimation of the rates of adverse reaction is much less important than the early detection of previously *unsuspected* adverse reactions. The emphasis is therefore on early identification on a qualitative basis. There have been a number of proposals but one obvious method is to permit normal launching and distribution of the drug and record in some way basic details of all those patients who receive the drug for whatever reason. Dovetailing in with the existing CSM's 'yellow-card' system (spontaneous reporting) once a serious reaction is signalled, it could then be checked or looked for in all of the other patients receiving the drug. In addition, all could be routinely checked at intervals of, say, one year, which would mitigate the drawback of under-reporting which the yellow-card system suffers from. One of the advantages of this is that cost is more closely related to benefit because it uses machinery already in existence, and since it would use large numbers of patients' records, even if only simply recorded, the chances of detecting a rare event would seem to be enhanced.

In the absence of fixed regulations requiring post-marketing surveillance, most companies have instituted varying degrees of monitoring on their own behalf. This has the advantage of indicating responsible attitudes, controlling costs to a degree (although these studies are expensive – a 3000–patient study would cost about £400 000) and giving a degree of international credence to the information generated.

The subject is an emotive and vexed one. Mild adverse effects (e.g. nausea) which occur commonly are no real problem. They are acceptable in the context of the treatment regime. The difficulty is the severe side-effect (sometimes fatal) occurring out of the blue in only a very few cases, often afflicting young adults who have not themselves previously been suffering from a life-threatening condition. Such events catch the headlines and give rise to much adverse undeserved publicity. The difficulty of the task may be appreciated if one considers an event which occurs at 1 in 50 000 (e.g. aplastic anaemia with phenylbutazone); one would need 1 570 875 patient years of follow-up to detect it accurately.

As already observed, the most important factor in adverse-reaction monitoring is undoubtedly the attending physician. His vigilance and perspicacity are irreplaceable and, coupled with skilled co-ordination between himself, company medical advisers and representatives, harm to individuals can either be minimised or prevented altogether. When one considers the variety of different therapies many such patients are taking, coupled with the onward march of their pathologies and the complexities of life (diet, etc), the difficulty of unravelling a suspected adverse reaction to the extent of strong probability (let alone absolute proof) can be appreciated. Proof is really only forthcoming if it is possible to rechallenge the patient with the suspected offending agent. For a variety of ethical and other reasons this is usually just not possible. From another more radical standpoint, careful investigation is nonetheless important, since it should not be forgotten that today's adverse reactions, no matter how bizarre, may open up avenues of research leading to possible cures of conditions that have barely been tackled.

Thus the post-marketing development phase is an important one in terms of continuing to define more closely the risk–benefit ratio in the mainstream indications and target population for which the registration of the new drug has been applied. Apart from this important and time-consuming aspect of adverse-reaction monitoring, the company will be mounting a variety of other studies, both clinical and non-clinical.

ADJUNCTIVE CLINICAL STUDIES

The two ancillary target populations of the young and the old have already been mentioned briefly. Perhaps the disease area that the new medicine is intended for is one which appears after childhoold has passed. If not, then this particular population will be specifically and sympathetically investigated. As we have seen, the elderly have problems associated with reduced absorption of drugs, slower drug metabolism and less-efficient excretion by kidney and liver. Taken together with differences in target organ sensitivity (the ageing brain and the decline in autonomic nervous system function), the problems of clinical trial in this particular group can be envisaged. Additionally, this group has generally lost what most other groups still have – a steady state of health – they are more prone to intercurrent illness and can withstand it less well. The elderly are more sensitive to heat and cold. They become a much less homogeneous group. In parallel with all this, and perhaps not unexpectedly, they also suffer from adverse reactions to medications more frequently.

Apart from studies in different population groups such as the young and the old, inter-racial differences are now known, not only with regard to disease natural history and response to therapy but also with regard to differences in drug metabolism. As mentioned before, differences in drug metabolic response are also encountered *within* populations. As clinical research is nowadays an increasingly international discipline, the reactivity of such groups to the new medicine must be investigated in practical terms.

To have obtained registration of the drug initially, the company will have done clinical work to show how the new medicine stands in the light of the available competition. Trials will certainly have been done using the main target population and by comparing the new agent with the established 'market leader' both comparative efficacy and also adverse reactions will be studied. However, nowadays there is often a series of important competitive agents which, in an effort to profile further the new agent commercially, will have to be investigated. Often by this process the range of indications is increased.

DRUG INTERACTION

Because patients who are ill in varying degrees are not taking a single medication but several, the question of drug interaction becomes important. Therefore the compatibility of the new therapy with other concomitant therapies must be checked. They need not be deleterious; often drug interactions are beneficial. The number of drug interactions is considerable which is not surprising considering the size of the present-day therapeutic armoury. One medicine can delay absorption of another (e.g. the tricyclics which alter gastro-intestinal tract mobility). They can compete for serum protein binding sites (Phenylbutazone and Warfarin) or for receptor sites (Phenothiazines and acetyl choline). Metabolism can be altered (barbiturates and enzyme induction) or renal metabolism can be altered (Probenecid – this is one which can be used to prevent the too rapid excretion of penicillin). More importantly, even latent pre-existing disease can be unmasked and exacerbated often with very serious results (steroid drugs and TB). Sometimes if the drug is to be given by injection it can react physically with other injections so that either potentially harmful solid matter is formed which blocks the needle, or the new drug may be so altered in character that it is not bioavailable to the body.

MISUSE AND ABUSE

Other aspects which must be investigated, depending on the nature of the agent, are such factors as over use, misuse and abuse liability. The latter is particularly true of some analgesic agents which *parri passu* with conferring effective analgesia may also produce pleasant feelings of well being. This will clearly lead to the drug being sought after by individuals for these reasons rather than for its analgesic properties. It is now usual to test these agents in this respect before registration is granted. This is a very specialised area and various sophisticated experimental procedures employing monkeys and other species are used which can give very sensitive indications of a compound's propensities in this direction.

However, it is possible for an experimental false negative to be recorded. If this is the case the potential of the new medicine in this respect will need to be established in intact man.

NEW FORMULATIONS AND PRESENTATIONS

During this phase the need for other formulations of the product may have become apparent. In this respect the project will 'revert back to the drawing board' to a certain extent, since a formulation will have to be designed and devised and then tested for reproducibility, scale-up, stability, etc. Examples could be an ointment or cream, or perhaps ear or eye drops, or even an injectable form. It may be that the original formulation, say a tablet, is not well accepted and the marketing department wants to change to a capsule. If this were the case then specific bio-equivalence studies directly comparing the new formulation with the old formulation would have to be performed on volunteers. In many of these instances further clinical work would, of course, be necessary.

When a new medicine becomes available for use in a larger patient population a number of poor responders, or even non-responders, may be identified. The reason for this must be established since it may yield new insights into the disease process itself, which again could give a pointer to further basic research and the possible creation of a new lead.

ADMINISTRATION DURING PREGNANCY

Often, despite warnings to the contrary, it is the nature of human life that the drug will eventually be administered to women who will be pregnant. This will often happen inadvertently and gives rise to a most difficult decision. If it is discovered early in the pregnancy, the usual answer is to remove the developing foetus. However, if it is not realised until later in the pregnancy and a scan shows an apparently normal baby, the decision may be taken to proceed to term. Careful documentation of the facts surrounding the case, coupled with the delivery of a normal infant, will be valuable in increasing knowledge and experience with the new drug. It is often by this process that knowledge is gained. Again the drug may be given in late pregnancy, e.g. an analgesic, and under carefully monitored and controlled conditions the effects on the foetus following delivery (by APGAR scores) can be defined. Furthermore, effects on breast feeding and whether or not the new drug is excreted in the milk could also be studied.

So far all the work in this post-registration phase has really been directed towards 'getting to know the compound better', i.e. exploring the major indications in different population groups and for longer periods of time. It has sought to quantify ever more exactly the risk–benefit profile both from the point of view of comparative therapeutic efficacy and adverse reaction incidence, type and quality. Another major area of investigation is that of indication development. Remember that the major indication was chosen in the first place on the basis of chemists' and pharmacologists' views of what the compound ought to do and what it ought to be good for. As a result of careful observations and further work during clinical research and development, the potential for investigation into other conditions or disease areas may arise. Sometimes this occurs late in development and is part of the post-registration development for many years.

INDICATION DEVELOPMENT

Quoting just two examples, figure 47 shows schematically the development of a minor tranquilliser while figure 48 shows the progress of an anti-dysrhythmic agent over time. With both drugs the dosage and the time to maximal response and the adverse effects to be expected at those dosages will already be known. With the development of different indications, problems may arise if the dosages necessary for treatment of those indications are greater than those where experience is already established. If such is the case, the work already described will need to be repeated since it will be breaking new ground and new adverse-reaction profiles may become apparent. Each new indication becomes a sub-project of the main one, at least at first, because the revenue potential for the second or third indication might eventually be hugely in excess of the original.

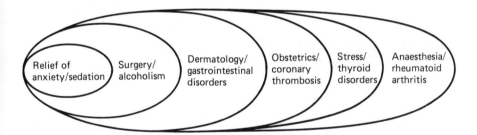

Figure 47 Showing the development of a minor tranquilliser used in different areas of medicine.

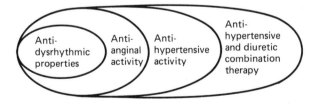

Figure 48 Showing the process of indication development, spanning several years, associated with a cardiovascular drug.

Company medical advisers, marketing people, physicians in practice, etc can all contribute to this process. The one thing it needs is an original mind to give inspiration, together with the ability to co-ordinate effectively. Chance favours the prepared mind and it is surprising how often a new indication will arise from a chance observation.

This process of development and indeed interest in the product will go on for as long as it is used by man. Knowledge is never complete. New claims are always being made. As each new claim is proved it has to be registered. However, as total experience with the new medicine is constantly accumulating, the process of registration may get easier for each new claim or indication.

13
International Development

The vast majority of new medicines have been, and are, developed by pharmaceutical companies. With the growth of excellent communications and fast international travel since World War II, the world has become in many respects a more unified entity. Science has really always been international but until about 25 years ago there was a tendency to develop drugs in the country where a company had its research and development facility, purely for the use of that indigenous population. If it was successful, then various forms of licensing arrangements were made with companies in other territories to develop it further and to exploit the medicine there. Essentially this was an inward looking and chauvinistic type of approach but, because the UK and other European markets needed to expand and the Americans wished to enter Europe, the pharmaceutical industry (being mainly either European or American) effected a transition to international activity. Of course, added to this there was also the influence of European firms in the countries of the old empires, and after World War II Japan increasingly came to be recognised as an international country in the pharmaceutical sense.

As a result of this, the post-registration phase in, say, six or seven countries is proceeding simultaneously with a pre-registration phase in a number of others. However, within the limits of cash resources the objective of good international development is to arrange the pre-registration development work on an international basis so that registration can be applied for virtually simultaneously in a number of important territories. Some companies are able to do this, others waste time and effort in not having matters properly co-ordinated. It is an important area because it is perhaps more 'controllable' than some of the other processes in R & D.

In order to maximise returns in this international arena the company has to anticipate where its largest opportunities may lie, since years in advance this assessment must be made in order to determine which territories should be the subject of patent application for the new invention. In some countries the degree of protection or exclusivity afforded is better than in others. The aim is usually to apply for patent protection as late as possible commensurate with ensuring that protection is not lost. The reason for the perhaps rather curiously worded 'as late as possible' is that once a patent application is submitted, the clock starts running, and there is a pressing need to push the project to registration as fast as is humanly possible because only then will the company have the longest equity life for its new invention. Again the submission (and probably also the granting of) patents will ideally need to be simultaneous in the priority countries. This aspect requires careful attention and often it suffers from a dearth of good planning activity. There are now many complaints about the amount of registration material which it is required to present to the national authorities. There are questions about its relevance and utility. It has been mentioned earlier that many of these factors are true and certainly have eroded the patent life of many medicines. However, the problem of maximisation of return on investment is often compounded by companies themselves in their not appreciating the need for planning and good timing in this area. Often because of vested interest, the pace is that of the slowest territory rather than the converse. In ideal circumstances efforts should be geared towards achieving more uniformity of patent and registration submission. Inevitably it must be a continuum, but should be over three to four years rather than ten years or more.

PATENTS AND TRADE-MARKS

Because patent applications are expensive it is usual for a company to have a policy whereby some countries are in a 'first division' for initial applications, followed by others in a second and even a third. In some countries there is no patent law and in others they are not worth applying for since the laws are not enforced.

Another important but perhaps less esoteric area than patents is that of trade-marks. Particularly in days of increased international activity when patients often travel round the world and expect to be able to obtain their medicines in the different territories they visit, it is much less confusing if the name of the product is the same or very similar in most territories. It is not as easy as it sounds since many companies over the years have built up banks of names which they own as industrial property. On the other hand, there could be similarities in trade-names devised for very different therapeutic areas. This is clearly undesirable since it will lead to confusion and enhance the possibility of mistakes on the part of both individuals dispensing medicines and those taking the medication. For this reason the authorities will not allow certain applications for trademarks because of a similarity to one already owned by another company. By the same token, a company may object to the granting of a trade-name to another company if it considers it is so close to one of their own trade-marks as to create confusion. A third problem area is where a perfectly good tradename in one territory has unfortunate connotations in another. For all of these and other reasons a company may set out to get the same trade-mark for its product in its major territories of operation but be frustrated in its efforts. However, with the exception of the linguistic difficulties already mentioned, companies do start searches and lodge applications for suitable trade-marks long before they are required. These form trade-mark banks and can give the company a slight advantage in that they have something to trade if another company has a trade-mark that they would like.

The increasing need for internationality of patents and trade-marks and registration relating to medicines, no matter which country they were originally invented in, in order to increase the chances of a suitable return for the years of investment in R & D, has therefore been explained. It may be that the company is not big enough or does not consider that it has the appropriate marketing structure to capitalise on its newly registered invention. For this and other reasons the cross-licensing of medicines has been developed to increase the chances of commercial success. Thus, for example, a company which is a market leader in the USA but which has no marketing presence in the UK, licences a drug to a British company to enable them to sell it for them for a return of a percentage of the revenue generated. Conversely, a British company may licence a drug to an American company for similar development. Sometimes such arrangements work well, but sometimes they founder for a variety of reasons, such as lack of commitment (NIH — not invented here), lack of understanding of what the originating company wants, etc. For these and other reasons most companies seem to have pursued courses where they have their own operations in the various territories of commercial interest to them. Because of differences in national attitudes and objectives, even this type of arrangement can have its difficulties.

Whatever the difficulties, the object is simple. Having invented, patented and started to develop a medicine in whatever country the R & D establishment is located in (sometimes there are more than one and this can indeed bring in other problems usually arising out of which particular novel product the company as a whole should progress), the essential step is to maximise the development pathway to achieve as near a simultaneous development as is possible in the group of territories that the company considers is most important to it. Different regulating authorities appear to slow up the development (or availability) process to different degrees (and the Food and Drug Administration — the FDA — is often cited here), but to this regulatory process must also be added the pharmaceutical industries' own 'drug lag'.

THE EXPANSION OF INFORMATION

Having said this, however, the problem is not a simple one. For a start, over the last twenty years or so the pharmaceutical industry has had to become adept at handling vast amounts of paper and vast amounts of data. This has led to the development of the discipline of information specialists in a number of different areas.

Initially pharmaceutical companies housed small libraries receiving and holding journals on chemistry, pharmacology, medicine and a few other disciplines

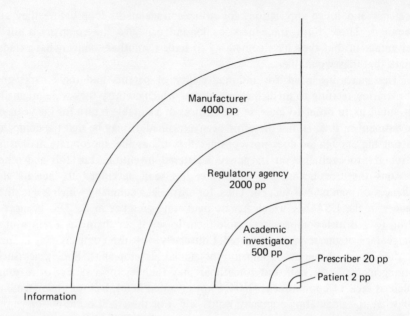

Figure 49 A diagrammatic representation of the information required for different purposes. During the course of development vast amounts of information are distilled down so that only information essential to correct prescribing is delivered to the doctor. Of course any further information required by individual doctors is readily supplied. (From Herxheimer, in *The Scientific Basis of Official Regulation of Drug Research and Development*, 1978.)

supplemented by a variety of textbooks. Over the last decade particularly, the number of journals has increased almost exponentially and this has also been accompanied by an explosion in the availability of books. Because the availability of knowledge and awareness of current activity in a whole variety of fields is the life-blood of the pharmaceutical industry (as, of course, with other industries), libraries had to expand rapidly to cope with this situation. Not every library can stock everything, but they must employ contacts with other information institutes to make sure that virtually every information request, no matter how seemingly bizarre, can be fulfilled reasonably quickly. This demand for increase in library space developed so rapidly at one stage that companies were rapidly running out of places to put books, periodicals, etc. Of course, necessity is as always the mother of invention, with the result that computer indexes with resultant capacity to do computer searches soon became available and much in-house information became stored on microfilm.

So far we have looked at the interaction of information between scientists of many different disciplines in an R & D department and activity outside it in thousands of centres around the world. But what about the corpus of information held within a company on its own products, product candidates, research lines, etc? Some of this will be published but a great amount will remain unpublished and will be in the form of internal reports and memoranda. Such information, if it is to be useful, must be entered into a system from which it can be retrieved. Whereas some years ago this might have been done by a simple card system, this has now progressed to become computerised.

Every time that a toxicology experiment, for example, is carried out, literally thousands of discrete pieces of information ranging from data on animals' statistics (weight, length, age, etc) through to behaviour observations and autopsy findings, are generated. All of these have to be entered into a system prior to analysis and report. When this sort of experiment is multiplied by all of those done in the other disciplines such as pharmacology, formulation development and clinical research, some idea of the complexity of the problem is gained. Most pharmaceutical companies now own their own powerful main-frame computer, usually connected to other big computers in other countries and fed by a number of terminals located throughout the establishment.

COMPUTERS

In parallel with this development, therefore, is the establishment of specialised computer personnel throughout the company. Prior to about 1970 it was relatively rare for a clinical-trial record form to be computerised, but as the need arose to examine more data points for more and more patients, literally the only way it could be successfully handled was to computerise the form at the input stage. (Initial attempts were made to make existing forms computer acceptable, but it was soon realised that unless the computer programmer had considered the matter before the fact as a specialist, there were invariably more problems than solutions by this method.) Obviously the manner in which questions are asked can have a material bearing on how they are answered, and therefore on the quality of the data at the end. It is now usual for clinical-research forms, adverse-reaction recording, etc to be fully computerised.

STATISTICS

Another discipline to be rapidly incorporated into drug development since about 1970 is that of statistics. Many early clinical trials failed to answer the question originally posed in the protocol (thereby wasting both time and money) because the patient numbers were inadequate or were of the wrong type (wrongly selected). In the constant struggle to get at the truth, statisticians are now involved in the very early stages of clinical trial protocol planning so that at least the question it is required to answer is examined in detail before committing resources. When they perform their statistical analysis later — from which the definitive report will be written — there is at least a chance that the information will be relevant.

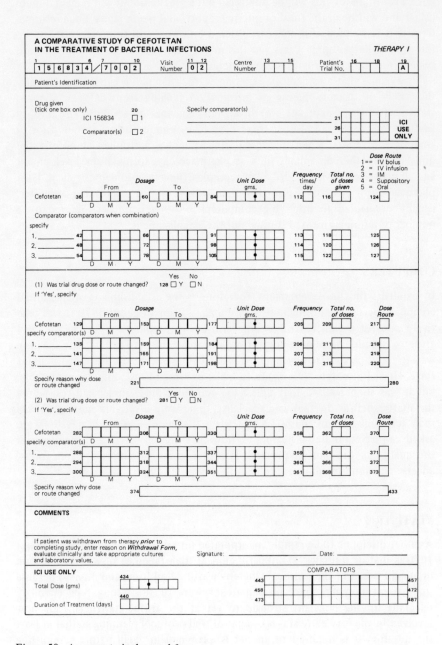

Figure 50   A computerised record form.

DATA EDITING

Of course, no matter how skilful and resourceful are the statisticians and computer programmers, the final common link in the quality of the data is that individual entering it on the record form (whether clinical or otherwise). Consequently, much time is expended in checking the records for errors, inaccuracies, omissions, etc before they are entered on to the computer. This painstaking work is performed by data editors. Wherever possible it is desirable to do this within the country generating the data since further problems could arise from language (semantic) difficulties and differences in national culture.

Originating before, but now certainly gathering pace in this field of international development, is the accumulation of a vast data bank on the new medicine. This data bank will be set in the context of the 'competition' as a world scene, both in terms of what is concurrently existing and in what likely developments may arise over the following months and years. This data bank is critical in terms of continuing to monitor the progress of the new medicine, from both the adverse reaction and efficacy standpoints.

PUBLICATIONS

During the course of an R & D programme a large number of scientific papers and communications will be prepared and submitted for publication. These papers are an important source of information for a company to gauge what areas its competitors are working in, and to be aware of what progress is being made. For this reason most companies have a system for checking material 'in house', e.g. its effect on patents, etc before submission to a journal, while others have a distinct policy, particularly in the clinical disciplines, of publishing material on a set plan. Obviously such a publication policy can ensure that competitors are not alerted too early, but at the same time it allows individuals to build their scientific reputations in tandem with company interests and objectives.

14
Risk − Benefit Ratio

The process of R & D so far described, which converts a chemical idea into a useful new medicine, is not a mechanistic one. It is not like a sausage machine where meat is put in at one end with complete and wholesome looking sausages issuing forth from the other. In the development of drugs there is no guarantee of success and when success is obtained it is usually the result of effective planning, great amounts of expended nervous energy and, of course, old fashioned good luck.

All drug development is now really directed towards forming as accurate an estimation as possible of the risk-benefit ratio from three major points of view − the government of the territory, the patient and the company − and to a certain extent, because the patient is not directly represented in the process, it comes down to a dialogue between the company and various government agencies in order to ensure that the patient is best served. It is in the interest of neither to ignore or minimise consideration of the patient's best interest.

If one goes back a few hundred years and beyond, the situation was much more simple. People were either healthy or ill, and those who were ill either got better or died. However, either those who were ill, or else their relatives, consulted others whom they believed could either reverse the situation or at best ameliorate it. The early practice of medicine was therefore based on the tenet that 'doing something was better than doing nothing'. Sometimes, however, in doing something the unsuccessful doctor suffered the same fate as his patient!

Gradually, as we saw in chapter 1, this process of empiricism did identify a number of agents which were beneficial in a number of disease states. However, a number of unsuccessful outcomes obviously occurred before the correct conclusions were drawn. In most developed countries there followed an early phase of legislation which tried to ensure that the public got value for money in the medicines it purchased, by setting penalties for the compounding and selling of quack medicines. (For instance, in England there was an act of 1540 which allowed for the appointment of four inspectors in London to control the quality of dispensed medicines.) From that time further legislation was directed against adulteration of drugs.

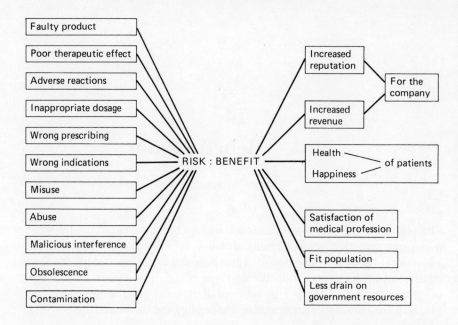

Figure 51 Some risks and benefits associated with the development of pharmaceutical products.

Certainly over the years, government control through various acts and regulations has become very sophisticated and thorough with regard to control of the quality of the medicine supplied. As an extension of the early acts in virtually all countries, a system of inspection of factories has been set up and is operated. This ensures that the quality of the ingredients and the standard of the process of manufacture is the highest possible attainable. Most countries have a system of Good Manufacturing Practices (GMPs) which ensure the highest quality from the beginning of the process until the material leaves the factory.

As an extension of this desire for the requisite quality and in response to problems over recording of experimental data, these regulations have in effect been extended into the area of good laboratory practice to ensure that the data produced at different stages during the years that the new medicine is undergoing development retain validity and are traceable to original sources. In addition various codes of conduct are now in existence for clinical practice also so as to ensure standardisation of procedures and production of data.

But government agencies did nothing to create any criteria of safety or efficacy until relatively late in the twentieth century when the events arising from Thalidomide administration in early pregnancy came to public notice. Governments then responded in an attempt to prevent the recurrence of such a tragedy by passing 'control of medicines' legislation which has been built-up considerably since the time of Thalidomide by additional regulations. All of it

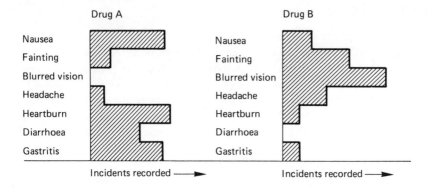

Figure 52   Two different adverse reaction profiles are shown, both obtained from, say, a sample of 500 patients. It can be seen that the profiles of A and B are different. In drug A there is a preponderance of gastrointestinal effects, while drug B appears to exhibit a greater 'neurological-type' profile. Of course the above takes no account of the severity of the effects or whether indeed some patients reported more than one effect.

is directed towards ensuring that such tragedies are not repeated. But does it?

There has been a great deal of talking and writing in an attempt to gain insight into the role of the government agencies which control the availability of drugs in their territories. In effect this is an examination of one aspect of the risk-benefit ratio since one has to balance out the risks to the patient population who would receive the drug against the benefits which would accrue to the majority. Against this has to be placed the benefits to those who might have been adversely affected by the drug if it never became available, together with the risks to that part of the patient population who are denied access to the drug. It is a complex equation and one to which no answer exists even in retrospect, unless a massive, costly and time-consuming prospective study is organised and mounted which extends over a considerable period of time. Even then one is still not out of the wood since such a study would gobble up tremendous resources which could certainly have been put to more advantageous use elsewhere.

Nor is this a purely theoretical situation. Over the last fifteen years the system of drug regulation in the USA has been such that a drug lag between America and Western Europe has been created which has of course resulted in a 'drug lack'. As an example, protagonists of this drug-regulatory system have pointed to the fact that its extreme slowness in approving Practolol prevented injury (from the unwanted effects identified subsequently after regulatory approval in various countries in Western Europe) to a number of American citizens who might have been affected. What has not been quantified is the number of Americans who might have had their quality of life improved if Practolol had been made available, or indeed who might have been harmed in other ways by alternate medicines.

PREDICTABILITY

The problem is therefore one of predictability. If one could predict which patients would suffer an adverse effect, and if one occurred would it be severe and life threatening or mild and self-limiting, then the predictability puzzle would be solved. However, such is not the case. The regulatory requirement for two-species carcinogenicity studies does not guarantee that a medicine is safe from this standpoint, although it does exclude some. It is extremely doubtful as to whether it will ever be so, particularly because so much of the whole process is continually breaking new ground. It is not an ideal world, and the best that can be achieved is a reasoned approach.

Animal studies in pharmacology give the researcher a basis for his expectation, which is only confirmed or dismissed by performing the experiments on man. On the other hand, the toxicologist, using again perhaps imperfect models, seeks to provide his clinical colleagues with a degree of reassurance before the new medicine is given to patients. Clinicians, by ensuring that the best equipment is available together with appropriate specialist help, try to minimise the consequences of an unforeseen and drastic event. In fact, such dramatic events rarely occur as adverse reactions of this type are usually the most predictable. Throughout clinical studies, physicians are constantly monitoring patients to ensure that if something untoward should occur it is recognised and acted upon immediately.

EXPECTATION OF SAFETY

Undoubtedly based upon early successes such as penicillin, the public has come to expect effective medicines which are extremely safe. At the same time it appears to be expected that surgery (perhaps because of its more dramatic connotations) is attended by a degree of risk. Apart from this immediate risk, it is also becoming realised that certain surgical procedures, such as those done for duodenal ulceration, carry a small but discernible predisposing risk of subsequent cancer. However, it must be continually stressed that in therapeutics as in life itself there is no such thing as absolute safety for every individual or indeed absolute safety for the same individual at different times. Thus in a trial, a particular adverse reaction may affect a small and unpredicted percentage of a patient population but not the remainder. However, this does not mean that the remainder can continue to take the drug perfectly safely since there may be other adverse reactions appearing later which may be more serious. Similarly with medicines which are taken intermittently, they may be perfectly harmless in one, two or three administrations, and then be associated with an adverse reaction on the fourth occasion. This assessment of risk is absolutely crucial. If a drug is an effective therapy in a life-threatening condition, but is known on occasions to produce a very serious adverse effect (even death), it will clearly still be beneficial if the patient is likely to die in any case. On the other hand, if the condition is unpleasant but self-limiting (a cold, for example) any medicine which could produce a life-threatening adverse reaction is clearly unacceptable. Again, a drug which gives a number of adverse reactions (unpleasant but not necessarily very serious) will not be preferable to one where the incidence is much lower but the efficacy is equivalent.

RISK OF NON-AVAILABILITY

If the regulatory agencies were to pursue a policy of only allowing drugs to be registered which displayed a minimum of adverse reactions, the end result might therefore be a non-availability of medicines with all the concomitant harm that that might do, not only in the immediate term with regard to current drug development by industry, but also in the longer term where drug development would be made a less-rewarding business to be in in terms of return on investment. Innovation would then be stifled and with it the morale of research and development personnel. Such a policy would be to kill the geese that lay the golden eggs.

COMPENSATION FOR INJURY

If it is accepted that the risk of eliminating or minimising adverse reactions is not to create a situation of non-availability of drugs, then adverse reactions when they occur must be effectively handled by both the state (government regulatory agency) and the manufacturing company. West Germany and Sweden have a system of either insurance or strict liability of products causing injury (even if there is no evidence of a defect in the medicine) which does not preclude recourse under civil law against a manufacturer. Compensation, the maximum of which is strictly limited both for individuals and groups, is given for pain and suffering, disfigurement and other permanent injury, loss of income, cost of treatment, etc. There is a time limit for claims to be made and liability in Sweden ceases after fifteen years. A scheme with broadly similar aims has been enacted in Japan to compensate for injury due to adverse drug reaction. Most other countries rely on settling the matter under civil law alone. In effect, the concept of strict product liability has been substituted by regulations, and both governments (as the largest customers for medicines) and companies work together to ensure that risks, once identified, are effectively combatted and minimised and those injured (this also applies to clinical trials) are compensated. This is seen to be a more satisfactory outcome for the good of the majority of the population than preventing the availability of medicines. Adverse reaction is a development defect, not a manufacturing defect.

LACK OF EFFICACY

Earlier, in the marketing chapter, the impossibility of selling an ineffective drug, or one which had too great an incidence of adverse effects in relation to its efficacy, was commented upon. A medicine which does not fulfil its therapeutic promise is bound to fail. This is a risk to the company since it may well have expended some millions of pounds in development before it becomes apparent. However, in a free market-place there are often a number of different drugs which seemingly do more or less the same thing – these are the 'me-too' agents occasionally in the news. In fact, all of these medicines have broadly the same degree of efficacy although the precise population that they most suit may differ. They have differences in adverse-reaction profile, and over the course of time, as knowledge about them builds up, their relative profiles come into sharper focus. It is found that they may have particular utility in certain sub-populations or in certain situations. This is not the same as considering a potential new medicine which has lower efficacy and a worse adverse-reaction profile and incidence than the 'me-too' compounds mentioned above. The key to all these situations is knowledge which cannot be gained instantaneously. Certainly the more effective an agent is in relation to its adverse reaction profile the more successful it will be, and therefore the more cost-effective will have been the company's R & D, and the greater is the return on investment.

The pharmaceutical industry is both labour intensive, employing many highly paid specialists, and capital intensive. It is strongest in the developed western world where research into the prevalent western diseases is clearly the most interesting, and, if a good medicine is discovered, the most financially rewarding. It is for this reason that many companies are engaged in the same broad areas of research and development, with the result that a number of broadly similar medicines are registered for use. 'Broadly similar' does not mean precisely similar and, as noted above, most of these agents will find a specific therapeutic niche to fill. Often their true value in any field of therapy cannot be fully assessed until they have been in use for some years.

Although the majority of governments are concerned solely with safety and efficacy, some countries have become involved in the question of relative efficacy based upon the clinical-trial evidence presented to them. Sometimes compounds which appear similar to those already on the market may be denied access to that market on the grounds that there is no distinct additional utility. This can prevent the true worth of the compound becoming known, and indeed sharpens up the requirement of companies to be in the first two or three in the race, rather than, say, thirteenth. It is difficult to prognosticate on these matters, but as we have seen, although the risk–benefit ratio of such compounds may appear to offer no additional advantage, over the course of months or perhaps years this situation may alter and the denied medicine may become the treatment of choice for a certain condition.

UTILITY AND PRICE CONTROL

Governments are the pharmaceutical industry's largest customers and some seek to regulate the entry of products on to the market by consideration of the price they are prepared to pay for it or the level to which they are prepared to reimburse its cost to the patient. Once again, the company having expended perhaps millions of pounds in development, may find that the price granted to it makes it impossible to develop the medicine further.

There are therefore these two additional risks to the company. Firstly, that the government agency rejects the application for registration approval on the grounds of 'utility' or no especial advantage over medicines already available, or secondly, on price control. Both of these mechanisms may deprive a population of a potentially useful medicine, besides introducing further risks on top of the risks inherent in R & D to the company. This could be deleterious in the long run by inhibiting investment which would, in turn, slow down the availability of new medicines, constraining as it would investment in basic and applied science.

The assessment of the risk-benefit ratio is an area beset with all sorts of problems both practical, theoretical and ethical. The risk of a faulty product (for example, as in the case of a car with a badly designed braking system) can be almost eliminated in pharmaceuticals. Even if therapeutic efficacy could be guaranteed, what cannot be eliminated is the unpredictability of what will happen in toto to each and every patient to whom the drug is administered. This is the risk which must be accepted by society if science is to advance. By the same token, society must compensate those individuals who are so affected.

15

Integration and Innovation

Before World War II scientists in one country working on a particular discipline would be in contact with others similarly engaged in other countries. There was free interchange of information both by published and unpublished mechanisms which gave the cross-fertilisation necessary for an integrated approach, that is the facility to build upon ideas and experiences from different sources. This is now true for universities and other research institutions. It is much less so for the pharmaceutical industry because of the need to be ahead of the competition and to safeguard industrial property. As already described, most pharmaceutical companies operate a policy of vetting scientific papers and communications before they are submitted for publication in order to ensure that when a discovery is published it is either properly protected under patent law, or, by the time publication is approved it is not scientifically sensitive to the company. Inventions such as new compounds, etc are the subject of proper patent applications before publication is permitted. Nevertheless, researchers are encouraged to publish and to participate in the international scientific community by attending scientific meetings and discoursing with colleagues in other countries and companies. R & D is international – there are no borders for ideas or the solutions to problems.

Apart from this externalised scientific integration which usefully contributes to the germination and development of ideas, there is integration within the company itself. This is in terms of achieving development of a product suitable for human use in the shortest possible time commensurate with safety. Such is the role of project management but there are other ways in which integration can be critical to the development of new products.

TOXICOLOGY

It has already been shown that there are difficulties in predictability with some animal studies when extrapolated to man. These lie chiefly in the toxicological area, but also difficulties exist in some areas of pharmacology. Carcinogenicity testing is required whenever a compound is suspected of being potentially carcinogenic, is related to a known carcinogen or co-carcinogen, or is likely to

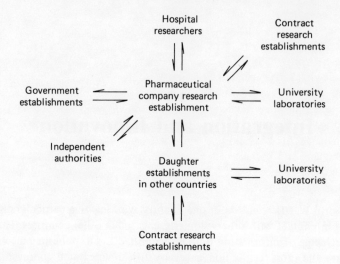

Figure 53 Showing some of the inter-related establishments in the scientific community which are involved in the cross-fertilisation and development of ideas.

be administered to man for period in excess of six months. Initially this was done in mice alone but is now extended to two species (rats and mice) and it will ensure that all those compounds giving a positive result will be excluded from long-term human administration. Even so, phenobarbitone for example is carcinogenic in rats but does not appear to be so in man. Among those giving a positive result in animals there might be extremely important compounds for the treatment of human disease which would not be investigated further. At the opposite end of the scale in this respect is the compound which is negative in animals but positive in humans. Because of the timescale involved and the numbers of certain cases which would be necessary to prove the case, these risks may never be quantified. In view of the long timescale and the expense of the life-time type of studies in rodents, various mutagenicity studies have been researched and promulgated. As with other animal manifestations of different toxicological profiles, it is necessary to try and relate these different effects to eventual outcomes in an effort to improve the state of the science. Thus the integration and free interchange of knowledge is necessary.

PHARMACOLOGY

The situation with pharmacology is similar to toxicology. Conditions like rheumatoid arthritis can be alleviated but the disease process itself cannot yet be either halted or reversed. The mechanisms whereby hypertension is mediated in different population groups are not yet fully understood, and although certain neoplasms have been successfully controlled, the rapidly dividing malignant cell has still not surrendered its secrets. However, the development of all the medicines since the 1950s, and in some cases before them, has enabled detailed studies to be made of their pharmacology with the result that further advances at the tissue-chemistry level have been permitted.

Because of the ever-escalating expense, a number of pleas have been made at least to reduce the costs per compound by permitting them to be used in man as soon as possible, so that those compounds which would fail on the grounds of lack of human efficacy could be terminated as soon as possible. This would free many clinicians and other workers to concentrate on those compounds which offered the best chance of future success. Relating such an event to the pharmacology just described would give scientists a chance to try and discover the reasons for the non-correlation of results. By this process of 'retrograde analysis' new and better predictors in animal tests could gradually be devised.

CLINICAL TRIALS

Clinical trials may be short and sharp in order to obtain an early view of efficacy and acute side effects (adverse or otherwise), but they must also be long term in an attempt to reveal long-term effects, both favourable and adverse. Of course, during this phase of development the observations of various clinicians are of importance since new, unsuspected and possibly extremely significant actions may be discovered. These are fed back from, say, the hospital clinician to the company's medical adviser and in turn to the medical adviser's pre-clinical colleagues. By this process, ideas and observations are integrated through the system.

Nor does it end there, because the same processes could be repeated with those involved with formulation development devising, on the basis of clinical observations, novel dosage forms or methods of administration. Suffice it to say that the whole process of constant feedback and integration is vitally important, not only for the new medicine under development, but also for new generations of products. By this process all personnel can and should have an input into the company's R & D programme in order to create new products and new techniques. For maximum effectiveness, they must be integrated with personnel from universities and research institutes with whom co-operation is very close.

16

The Organisation

The role of project management and its interlocking with product management has been examined. That an effective interlock exists is vital for the smooth transition of the new medicine from the R & D phase (i.e. pre-marketing) to the marketing phase. Since the product, unless it is withdrawn from the market for a particular reason, will always be the subject of some degree of investigation, these two key roles will co-exist for a very large part of the life of the new medicine – ideally for all of it.

R & D organisations, on the other hand, differ widely in structure, depending upon the type of company, its historical background and, most importantly, on the composition and capabilities of the personalities involved. It is labour intensive and is staffed by scientific specialists of high calibre.

An international organisation usually consists of both central and peripheral segments. The central part is where the main laboratory facility is sited. There may or may not be satellite research facilities elsewhere and the peripheral segment is composed of those small specialised units which have a direct involvement in the territories in which they are situated.

In any organisation, good communications and team spirit are essential, and this is particularly so wherever a geographically fragmented international organisation is concerned. Attention to this area by the company can do much to speed the development process relating to new medicines.

Essentially there are a number of main areas which will be briefly described in the order in which they become involved in the development process, although, as mentioned before, drug development is not strictly a linear process (see figure 55).

Discovery resides principally, but not exclusively, within two major departments. The chemistry department can be subdivided into research along specific lines of chemical synthesis investigation, analytical activity and techniques, and chemical process development. Accompanying this function is the biology department which subdivides into pharmacology (which itself is divided into teams investigating specific areas such as the cardiovascular system or central nervous system) and toxicology (with responsibility for the conduct of toxicity testing including housing and looking after what is usually a large animal population).

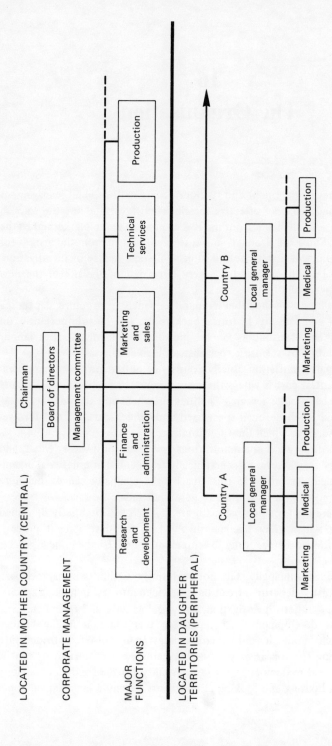

Figure 54   The central organisation located in the mother country (be it the UK, Germany, USA, Japan, etc.) controls the world-wide operation of the group in policy terms. Most organisations grant a significant degree of autonomy to their daughter organisations and affiliates, some of which may not be wholly owned.

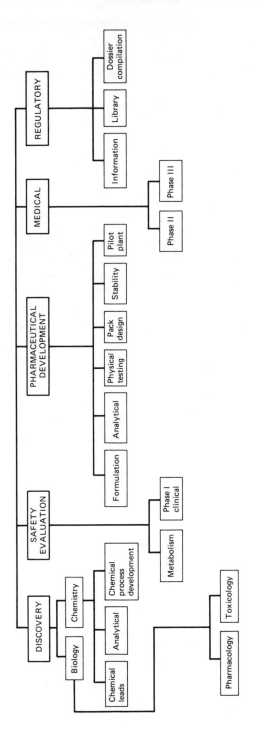

Figure 55

Safety evaluation, which may also include toxicology, is responsible for the metabolism work (absorption, distribution, metabolism and excretion) and leads on into human pharmacology or phase I clinical work. The results of these investigations will be fed back into animal pharmacology and forwards into clinical activity.

The next major division is that of pharmacy or pharmaceutical development. This function is usually subdivided into formulation studies, which is staffed by scientists who specialise in the creation of tablets, capsules, gels, creams, ointments, etc and produce formulations which will be specifically appropriate to the product under development. Others will be responsible for the physical testing and analysis of such formulations while the pack design and the stability of the whole product package will be initiated and followed by others. A pilot plant is usually included in a pharmaceutical development organisation since the behaviour of the new formulation on the machinery the company owns will need to be investigated before it is handed over to the production department.

Eventually the compound passes to clinical research which, by a careful stepwise incrementation, increases the patient population from a handful to perhaps 3000 or more as phase II and phase III clinical trials are initiated. It is usually at this stage that the satellite medical departments in various territories become involved as knowledge on international populations begins to be built up.

As we have seen, the regulatory affairs department, also consisting of skilled scientists, becomes involved once definitive data, which will be included in a submission to various national authorities, becomes available. These scientists have the responsibility of ensuring that the data are clear, concise, easily referable and, of course, meet the criteria required by the various national drug-regulatory agencies. Because of the necessity for handling large amounts of data, information and library services as a whole may be grouped in this department. Once all the appropriate preclinical and clinical information is assembled, it is paginated and bound into a regulatory submission and transmitted to national drug authorities. The amount can be enormous. Some submissions to authorities like the American Food and Drug Administration may comprise in excess of 250 weighty volumes of data.

Following the successful grant of a licence to market and distribute the product, the R & D department will still be involved in providing specialist help to physicians on how to use the product to best advantage and to do further (phase IV) clinical work. As we have seen, additional populations or indications are the subject of such work. In the main it is confirmatory, but is also in part innovatory. The company medical advisers involved in phase IV are also closely linked with the marketing function and participate in such important areas as representative training. In some companies they are organisationally a part of the marketing department.

Organisations are as many and varied as there are companies. Whatever the set-up the objective is to use the team to develop medicines in the shortest

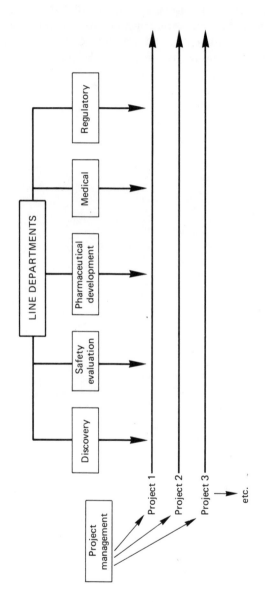

Figure 56

possible time, and project management therefore operates functionally across the line departments and can be represented as in figure 56.

The operation of project management across the line departments serves to illustrate that although the departments operate broadly sequentially, in actual fact the steps proceed at different rates for each project. It is the responsibility of the project manager to ensure that each particular project proceeds to completion in the optimum time.

17
The Future

The preceding chapters have attempted to describe, but only in the merest outline, the various processes which when skilfully fitted together result in the
genesis of a new medicine. It is a costly business in terms of time, money and
nervous energy. At innumerable points along the pathway a feedback-type of
activity is apparent where results and observations are constantly being compared with previous experience, in order to improve not only the actual process
itself, but also to identify ways to develop even better medicines in the future.
Research-based companies therefore compete through innovation to produce
better products and better techniques and they use this experience to open up
different research lines aimed even more specifically at the treatment and alle-
viation of a variety of disease states. In the main these disease states are those
which afflict the affluent western civilisations because the need to be successful
in a profitable area is paramount if more money is to be ploughed back into even
more R & D. Often though, discoveries are made which would beneficially affect
either rare conditions or 'third world' diseases such as various parasitic infesta-
tions. In the majority of instances development of such chemicals is not pursued
by the pharmaceutical industry because the difficulty of gaining registration,
together with the amount of work involved both before and after registration,
conspire to ensure that a reasonable return on the investment is impossible.
Sometimes organisations such as the World Health Organization or other interested bodies take on the responsibility for progressing these potential new
medicines. Usually, however, they rarely see the light of day. As previously
mentioned, the recent considerable increase in regulatory activity and the
requirements by governments around the world has had a number of deleterious
effects on innovatory R & D. For example, the number of new chemical entities
under development has recently diminished dramatically. In fact, to be specific,
it has been predicted that by the year 2000 they will have ceased to be developed
altogether if the present trend in regulatory activity is not reversed. This affects
not only the search for new medicines for 'western conditions' (because in any
R & D budget, diminishing quantities of money will be available for research),
but it also affects the development of medicines for 'third world' conditions
which companies will be increasingly unable to fund as a service because of the

cost of satisfying the regulations. The same arguments apply to medicines for rare conditions. For this reason they are often referred to as *orphan drugs*.

It may be counter-argued that companies are protected by the availability of patents, and under normal circumstances this would be true. However, regulatory delays in approving a new medicine continue to erode patent life with the result that the time available 'to replenish the treasury' is constantly diminishing. Apart from these external pressures, it is also true to say that inefficiency on the part of some companies in terms of effectively integrating their R & D activity on an international scale also leads to a loss of potential revenue. The most important factor in R & D is time, which once expended can never be replaced. In the process as a whole, events in development can be influenced in terms of time much more than those in research and it is in this area that increased efficiency must be obtained. Development, in effect, depends on economic calculation but with each step becoming more deliberate and being specifically designed towards a defined end. It is more controllable than research and great amounts of time can be saved by crisp and, to an extent, courageous, decision making coupled with effective integration and co-ordination of the development process. There is no such thing as instant R & D — it has to be preplanned.

SAFETY

The constant search for absolute safety has been likened to the pursuit of the Holy Grail. Because of the publicity which has surrounded a variety of untoward events since World War II, coupled with the fortuitous discovery of a series of comparatively very safe drugs, the public now expects better drugs and expects them to be extremely safe. Governments, as chief customers, expect cheaper drugs as a result of ever-present pressures on the public purse. It is in order to satisfy the expectation of safety that the elaborate regulatory activity already described has arisen. Many think that it has done little to increase public safety and has certainly made the prospect of cheaper innovations impossible.

STATE OF THE ART

Animals

All biological science suffers from various degrees of imperfection. In terms of toxicology the current emphasis is on quantity, coupled with long-term studies which in themselves have known limits in terms of the risks they will be able to identify (even if the animals should behave in the same way as man). It follows then that these studies should logically progress to research into the mechanisms of toxicity with the subsequent development of new models to improve predictability. By the same token, the science of teratology is beset with a relative lack of knowledge of the pharmacokinetics across the placental barrier, such as the dosage and timing of introduced substances which may be compounded by intercurrent maternal conditions. Efforts are continually being made to extend knowledge in these and other problem areas. Despite the fact that in 1981 some 4 300 000 animals were used in research (very many it is true to say, in minor and non-painful procedures not associated with pharmaceutical R & D) the state of the art is such that the abandonment of the use of animals is still a very long way away, and for a variety of good reasons. For instance, teratological experiments, whatever their present shortcomings, could not be replaced by tissue culture techniques because of cell chromosomal changes *in vitro*. This means that the same type of cell is not present throughout the experiment. Furthermore, techniques *in vitro* would give no information or input into the effect of new medicines on the physiology of the circulatory or excretory systems (liver, kidneys, etc), the brain, sense organs, lungs or alimentary canal. The same is true of carcinogenicity (lifetime) studies in both rats and mice which are now required for many new substances. They will detect, it is true, a carcinogenic risk of 3% but will not reveal a weak carcinogen in its true colours. Furthermore it is possible that effective medicines have already been lost to man if one considers that phenobarbitone (introduced long before carcinogenicity testing was even thought of) is significantly carcinogenic in one species of animal but presumably not to man. Under present-day procedures it would never gain regulatory acceptance.

So far the imperfection of animal studies as predictors of the toxicological behaviour of a new medicine in man have been briefly reviewed. Imperfect they may be, but at the moment it is all that is available. However, efforts are being continuously made to improve their predictability.

Man

In view of this situation the greatest step forward is the first administration to humans, which, as already described, is performed with 'eagle eyes and bated breath' by the clinical pharmacologist. This is the acid test because, even though the effects of the new medicine on the overall physiology of animals will already be known, the effects on humans may or may not be comparable. This is also true with regard to the early animal toxicology experiments. By gradually building up the dosage and then moving towards multiple dosing, the effects of the new substance are carefully monitored and the experience gained is cycled back to the research scientists. When the researchers are confident, and after regulatory approval in many territories, they are ready for that second great leap forward — trial of the new medicine in man with the pathology to be treated, influenced or cured — the patient. Whereas the human-pharmacology studies will have conferred confidence with regard to the absence of acute noxious physiological or toxic events, in the majority of R & D programmes information up to this point is pure supposition with regard to efficacy. Of course, there may be a strong supposition in many instances, but until the hurdle is actually jumped there is no certainty. The build-up of proof of efficacy has already been des-

The Development of a Medicine

Table 16.1

Rate of event per year of exposure	Relative risk	Required person-years of follow-up
1 : 500	200	3965
1 : 1000	100	8010
1 : 5000	20	43 495
1 : 10 000	10	96 929
1 : 20 000	5	245 376
1 : 50 000	2	1 570 875

cribed in both chapter 7 and in subsequent chapters. It continues for years and may extend into different indications. However, no medicine can reasonably be expected to be effective and at the same time completely free of side-effects. Some side-effects can be beneficial (e.g. a centrally acting (i.e. on the brain) anti-hypertensive agent which is also mildly anxiolytic), but the majority are unwanted or adverse. They range in severity from intercurrent nuisance value (e.g. nausea) to being life-threatening (e.g. anaphylactic reactions). This is where the problem lies — the expectation of absolute safety for each and every individual. It is clearly an unacceptable expectation, but even so, great efforts have been and are being made by a very large number of skilled individuals to research into ways of enabling a more accurate identification of those individuals at risk to be made, thereby minimising the impact of such unwanted effects. Where some are concerned (i.e. in-built deficiencies of oxidative or acetylative metabolism, or susceptible genotypes as evidenced by Hydrallazine and the systematic Lupus erythematosus syndrome), they can be identified by screening. The possibility of exposure to toxic events as a result can be eliminated. However, the vast majority of adverse reactions are initially unquantifiable, and it requires large numbers of patients to be studied, as table 16.1 (based on Shapiro's observations) indicates. In addition, at the moment it is not possible to predict in advance who will get the adverse reaction. However, current thinking is directed towards the objective that if adverse reactions can be identified early enough, the possibility exists that by immediately withdrawing the drug for those affected individuals, damage or injury will be minimised. In addition, if a large enough 'scan' of the 'at-risk' population is undertaken, it will enable a valued judgement to be made as to the degree of risk for that population. The UK's spontaneous reporting by the 'Yellow Card' system has already been alluded to. It was instituted in 1963, and despite the considerable drawback of under-utilisation (under-reporting), has given good service. The World Health Organisation (WHO) operates a similar system by compiling the national returns into an international register. More recently, Inman has proposed and carried into effect a Prescription Event Monitoring system which allows identification of doctors prescribing a new drug who are subsequently contacted to see if any unusual or untoward event has occurred. An adverse reaction can be detected against background noise by a follow-up (either regionally or nationally) of all those individuals who have received the new drug. As soon as an adverse reaction 'looms on the horizon' the full cohort of patients can be immediately checked to ascertain whether or not a problem exists. Furthermore, the incidence of such an adverse reaction can be gauged because the number of events (numerator) and number of patients (denominator) is known.

ADVERSE REACTION INVESTIGATION

Of course, the establishment of an adverse reaction as a true event may be far from easy. Companies, like governments, are concerned to get at the truth because, apart from the possible damage to patients, there is a risk of attendant loss of revenue, coupled with damage to their reputations. The company concerned will therefore go through an investigatory cycle of identification, validation, evaluation and explanation of the effect. The issue can be clouded by a similarity to a new or existing illness in the patient or the existence of interaction with other concomitantly administered medicines. Indeed, whether the new drug was properly prescribed against an accurate diagnosis and correctly dispensed by the pharmacist, and whether the patient took it as prescribed, will all have to be investigated before a judgement is made. In view of the obvious need for medical skill and judgement in this area, many companies employ one or more well-qualified physicians whose sole responsibility it is to monitor and evaluate all these reactions. An important task, because the true, serious adverse reaction may be very difficult to winkle out from the background noise of subjective and other complaints to which man is heir. No matter what system is employed, effective and sympathetic communication between all concerned is the essential component.

A consideration of adverse reactions, and it should be reiterated that the vast majority are either predictable as knowledge builds up, or else of no serious moment, reinforces one's realisation that safety is not, and can never be, absolute in each and every individual. However, with modern efficacious therapeutics, the benefits to the vast majority of people, and therefore to society, are enormous and at comparatively trivial financial cost per capita. Even the cost of a course of some of the most expensive modern advances is extremely small when compared with the expense of hospitalisation for two or three weeks, or that of a moderately complicated surgical operation. It does seem to be natural justice, however, that those individuals who have been injured as a result of an unlucky statistical or biological accident in the pursuit of an overall benefit to society should be appropriately compensated for their injury.

Considering R & D overall in the light of the great numbers of therapeutic agents which have been registered in the last three decades, it is apparent that drugs are in general remarkably safe in practical terms. The progress of successful medicines which eventually reach the therapeutic armoury has been described briefly. It takes no account of the 10 000 or more compounds which are examined and rejected in the search for each successful new medicine. This process might be considered wasteful but each one adds, however minutely, to the fund of knowledge or 'enabling science' on which the future depends.

It is hoped that the foregoing description of what is, after all, a very complex integrated process will have given the reader some insight into the overall responsible nature of the pharmaceutical industry. However, no matter how well it exercises that responsibility it will always be dogged by problems of safety for particular individuals because it operates at the 'cutting face' of new knowledge. To continue the analogy, every so often one inadvertently cuts into a new and unpredictable hazard, but this does not, and should not, deter man from fully continuing to explore his environment.

Bibliography and Suggestions for Further Reading

Cavalla, J. F. (ed), *Risk–Benefit Analysis in Drug Research*, MTP, (1981)

Dayan, A. D. and Brimblecombe, R. W. (eds), *Carcinogenicity Testing: Principles and Problems*, MTP (1978)

De Schaepdryver, A. F. *et al.* (eds), *The Scientific Basis of Official Regulation of Drug Research and Development*, Heymans Foundation, Ghent (1978)

Edwards, A. M. *et al.* (eds), *Drugs in Pregnancy, Paediatrics and Geriatrics*, The Trust for Education and Research in Therapeutics (1981)

Good, C. S. (ed), *The Principles and Practice of Clinical Trials*, Churchill Livingstone, Edinburgh (1976)

Harcus, A. W. (ed), *Risk and Regulation in Medicine – The Fettered Physician*, Association of Medical Advisers in the Pharmaceutical Industry (1980)

Inman, W. H. W. Various communications from the Drug Surveillance Research Unit, University of Southampton

Lahon, H. *et al.* (eds), *Pharmaceutical Medicine – The Future*, Acta Therapeutica, Brussels (1979)

L'Etang, H. (ed), *Regulation and Restraint in Contemporary Medicine in the UK and the USA*, The Royal Society of Medicine and Macmillan (1983)

Richards, D. J. and Rondel, R. K. (eds), *Adverse Drug Reactions*, Churchill Livingstone, Edinburgh (1972)

Robinson, R. G. (ed), *Therapeutic and Unwanted Effects: Drug Related or Not?*, Huber, Vienna (1977)

Teeling-Smith, G. and Wells, N. (eds), *Medicines for the Year 2000*, Office of Health Economics (1979)

International Drug Registration, IFPMA Symposium, Geneva. IFPMA, Zurich (1979)

Various ABPI reports issued 1975–1977, including: (1) *Bioavailability Studies in Drug Development.* (2) *Guidelines for Pre-clinical and Clinical Testing of New Medicinal Products.* Part 1: *Laboratory Investigations*; Part 2: *Investigations in Man.* (3) *The Report of the Committee to Investigate Medical Experiments on Staff Volunteers*

Wardell, W. M. and Lasagna, L., *Regulation and Drug Development*, American Enterprise Institute for Public Policy Research, Washington (1975)

Wells, N., *Medicines: 50 Years of Progress 1930-1980*, Office of Health Economics (n.d.)

Index